waiting to happen

waiting to happen

HIV/AIDS IN SOUTH AFRICA – THE BIGGER PICTURE

Liz Walker Graeme Reid Morna Cornell

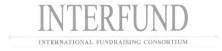

LYNNE
RIENNER
PUBLISHERS

boulder
london

Published in 2004 in the United States of America by
Lynne Rienner Publishers, Inc.
1800 30th Street, Boulder, Colorado 80301

and in the United Kingdom by
Lynne Rienner Publishers, Inc.
3 Henrietta Street, Covent Garden, London WC2E 8LU

and in Southern Africa by Double Storey Books,
a division of Juta & Co. Ltd,
Mercury Crescent, Wetton, Cape Town

ISBN 1-58826-263-4 (Lynne Rienner Publishers)
ISBN 1-919930-39-6 (Double Storey Books)

Design and layout by Jenny Sandler
Cover design by Toby Newsome
Printed and bound in the Republic of South Africa by Creda Communications,
Cape Town.

5 4 3 2 1

Library of Congress Cataloging-in-Publication Data
Walker, Liz.
    Waiting to happen : HIV/AIDS in South Africa : the bigger picture /
Liz Walker, Graeme Reid, and Morna Cornell ; with a foreword by Edwin
Cameron.
        p. ; cm.
Includes bibliographical references and index.
    ISBN 1-58826-263-4 (pbk. : alk. paper)
    1. AIDS (Disease)–South Africa. 2. AIDS (Disease)–Social aspects–South
Africa. 3. HIV infections–South Africa. 4. HIV infections–Social aspects–South
Africa.
    [DNLM: 1. HIV Infections–epidemiology–South Africa. 2. Acquired
Immunodeficiency Syndrome–epidemiology–South Africa. 3. Acquired
Immunodeficiency Syndrome–ethnology–South Africa. 4. HIV Infections–
ethnology–South Africa. 5. Social Problems–South Africa.
    WC 503.4 HU5 W181w 2003] I. Reid, Graeme. II. Cornell, Morna. III. AIDS in
    Context Conference (2001 : University of the Witwatersrand) IV. Title.
    RA643.86.S6W357 2003
    362.196'9792'00968–dc22
                                        2003023323

CONTENTS

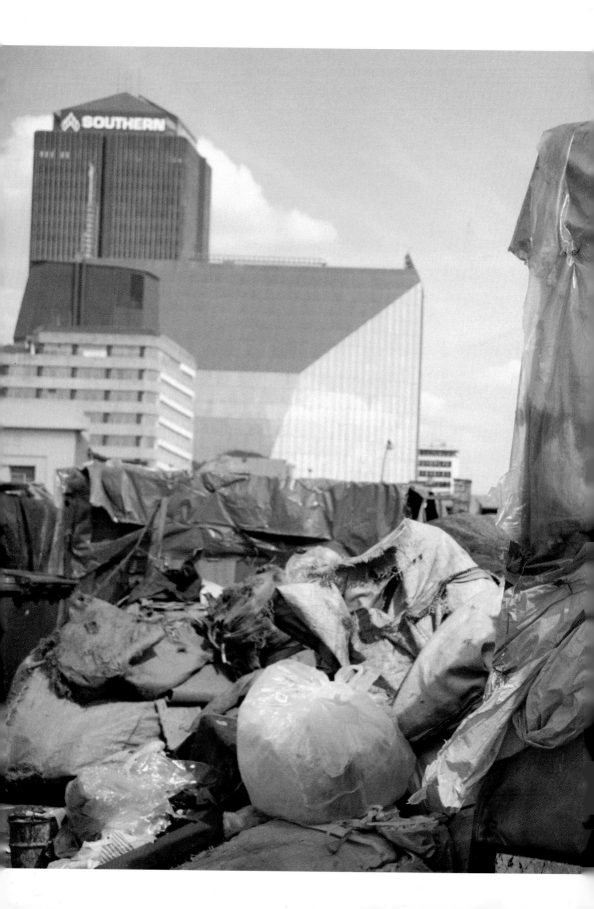

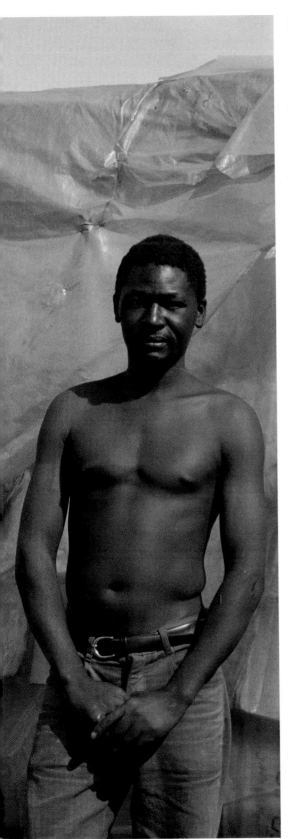

FOREWORD

Waiting to Happen: HIV/AIDS in South Africa emerges from 'AIDS in Context' – the most important national deliberative conference on AIDS thus far held in South Africa. The book draws on an impressive and authoritative range of papers that address the social, cultural and historical roots of the epidemic in a region heavily burdened by AIDS. It is therefore published at an acute time.

AIDS has from the outset been as much a battle of ideas as a battle about bodies and organisms and cells. From the start, the disease was stigmatised, its first known bearers being the gay men of the west and east coasts of America, of London and Paris, and of Sydney, Johannesburg and Cape Town. Thereafter, it was associated with stigmatised minorities in the United States and elsewhere. The momentous demographic difference between the first diagnosed case of AIDS in June 1981 and the present is, of course, that the disease now overwhelmingly affects poor heterosexuals in the developing world.

What these groups have in common in their vulnerability to AIDS is that it remains overwhelmingly a disease of the marginalised and the stigmatised and, in Africa, of the dispossessed. Of all the desolate figures and statistics that this epidemic presents, none is more awesome than that two-thirds of all those living with HIV and AIDS in the world are in Sub-Saharan Africa; and that 90% of them are in the developing world.

Those figures starkly mirror the more general disparities in our world between those who control and those who do not; between those who have taken possession and those who have been dispossessed; those who have, and are surrounded, and are well attended, and those whose circumstances are the opposite. AIDS therefore mirrors, but it also accentuates, the disparities of our world.

It does so in a particularly dramatic way. A more dramatic change than that of demography is that AIDS no longer has to be a fatal illness. Life-saving combinations of anti-retroviral drugs have shown that illness and death from AIDS can be contained. Under the right conditions, HIV is now a chronic, manageable infection, and AIDS a treatable disease.

'The right conditions' include adequate medical care and attention, basic nutrition, monitoring of drug and viral levels in the blood, and, most imperatively, access to the new combination drug therapies.

It is this last condition that has formed the focus for public debate about and public response to the epidemic in the recent past. It is right that this should be so. The disparities between First and Third Worlds are masked by structure and distance and the global status quo of commodity prices and debtor–creditor relationships. In all of this, charges of injustice and exploitation can be refuted all too glibly.

But the calculus of disease and death from AIDS renders the self-serving rhetoric dramatically unconvincing. None of it is persuasive when the brute fact is accepted that life is available and within reach, but is being withheld from those who crave it by pricing structures and policies, and by governmental ineptitude and lack of political leadership.

It is in this context that the empowerment of people living with HIV and AIDS takes on a particular significance. The Treatment Action Campaign (TAC) has at every level dramatically changed the terms of the debate about AIDS in South Africa. It has revived a dispirited movement amongst persons living with AIDS by giving them dignity in hope and action. It has through information and argument shifted the terrain on which the debate about denial of medications is taking place.

More broadly, the TAC has reminded all South Africans of the importance of strategic and principled activism, built upon effective alliances, in pursuit of elementary justice for those denied it. In recognising this we salute our own history as South Africans, but we also look ahead to what we ought yet to achieve as a nation.

It is precisely through activism that persons living with HIV and AIDS have reclaimed their own destiny – not as 'sufferers' or 'victims', but as human beings with a right to live, in a world that can afford the material conditions to realise that right.

By that act of reclamation and self-assertion, the argument against the effective administration, supervision and monitoring of medications is refuted. It is in part by according people living with AIDS and HIV the dignity, the capacity and the power to assert themselves as human beings that we create the conditions for effective drug administration and thus the containment of the disease.

This epidemic has been a battle of ideas in which the activist assertion of ideals has started to reclaim the fundamental entitlements of life.

The battle for treatment access has also refuted another damaging and disempowering rhetorical divide. Too often we have been told that prevention is more important than treatment; that the only effective way to counter this epidemic is to concentrate on the uninfected; and that those already infected must be left to face their fate with what sympathy and support our already overstretched resources can muster.

The dichotomy is false. Physiologically, treatment is a form of prevention. This is most dramatically evident in mother-to-child prevention programmes, where administering drugs to a mother in parturition has a good chance of preventing transmission to her baby. There is also good physiological evidence that an effective course of anti-retroviral medication prevents or substantially inhibits sexual transmission of the virus.

Psychologically, treatment also enhances prevention, since it affords those already infected with a dramatic incentive to come forward to be tested, to receive counselling, and to engage fruitfully with the complexities of behaviour modification. The evidence from poor rural and urban areas in Africa is already powerful. Pilot projects on mother-to-child transmission offering voluntary testing to women presenting at an antenatal clinic result in dramatically increased uptake of HIV testing.

But, third and most important, treatment also enhances prevention socially. By treating people we offer them hope. And by offering hope in this epidemic, we dispel the notion that AIDS is hopeless, that it is fraught with failure, and that once infected the subject can face only debilitation and death.

Treatment has irreversibly broken the equation between AIDS and death. By this breakthrough, we can begin to undo the social stigmas and phobias that make prevention so difficult to talk about frankly.

We are burdened by a national prevalence that, translated into percentages or absolute numbers in millions of South Africans, defies acceptance and belief. We have been burdened by governmental failings before and after our transition to democracy, in which ineptitude on the part of the apartheid government in dealing with AIDS has been grievously matched by our democratic government.

Thirty-five million people in the developing world face death – a cruel and lingeringly debilitating death – unless we are impelled to action. The actuaries and the statisticians make an unanswerable case that the next decade will see tens of millions of deaths unless we intervene.

And one thing is incontestably clear. We have the means to intervene. In my own life I have been able to change the imminent prospect of death from AIDS. My life has the attributes of love and protection of family, friends and colleagues; security and engagement of work and involvement; and access to life-saving medications. Without those conditions, I would quite simply not be alive. These we ought to be committed to extending to everyone affected by this epidemic.

I cannot claim life for myself without asking why others, no differently placed except for the happenstance of affluent connection, should face debilitation and death. None of us can.

This remains the central challenge of AIDS today. Our response to it will determine our place in history as activists, as intellectuals, and indeed as people.

Mr Justice Edwin Cameron
Supreme Court of Appeal
10 May 2003

PREFACE

Social scientists have been slow to respond to the HIV/AIDS epidemic. Studies have either been too general or have focused on one community. There is a limited understanding of the social factors that have fuelled the epidemic. The immediacy of the epidemic and the urgent pressure for solutions to this enormous problem have meant that much social science research has been either superficial or epidemiological in nature. This pattern has often been shaped by donor agencies that have been equally determined to find a quick-fix solution. Thus the demands of the epidemic have meant that there has been little time for considered, long-term, social-scientific research and analysis. Much work remains to be done on the social dynamics of HIV/AIDS.

It was in recognition of these factors that the AIDS in Context Conference took place at the University of the Witwatersrand, Johannesburg, in April 2001. Academics, researchers and AIDS activists took part in a rich and varied programme. Over a hundred papers were presented, highlighting new and diverse material. Panel discussions and plenary sessions also enriched the conference. The material for this book has largely been drawn from this conference. We hope that we have captured some of the texture and diversity of the research and ideas presented there. We would like to thank all the conference participants who made their papers and presentations available for use in this publication.

The conference was a joint initiative of the Wits History Workshop, the Centre for Health Policy (School of Public Health, University of the Witwatersrand), Soul City, the AIDS Consortium, and the Gay and Lesbian Archives of South Africa. Ralph Berold and Simonne Horwitz organised it with tireless enthusiasm.

The production of this book has been a collective effort. Philip Bonner, Peter Delius, Helen Schneider and Sally Ward of the AIDS in Context organising committee played a key role in conceptualising and structuring the book and provided insightful commentary on drafts of chapters throughout. Morna Cornell made a significant contribution to the broader project by organising the material and working on the initial manuscript. Rita Potenza of South Photographs sourced the images for the book and Margaret Ramsay did the final language edit.

The conference was funded by Atlantic Philanthropies, Anglo American/TSI, Soul City, the University of the Witwatersrand Research Office, and the University of the Witwatersrand Faculty of Humanities. Generous grants from Interfund and Atlantic Philanthropies ensured the publication of the book. Special thanks go to Gerald Kraak of Atlantic Philanthropies and Riana Botes of Interfund.

The Wits Institute for Social and Economic Research (WISER) has provided invaluable institutional support.

Liz Walker and Graeme Reid

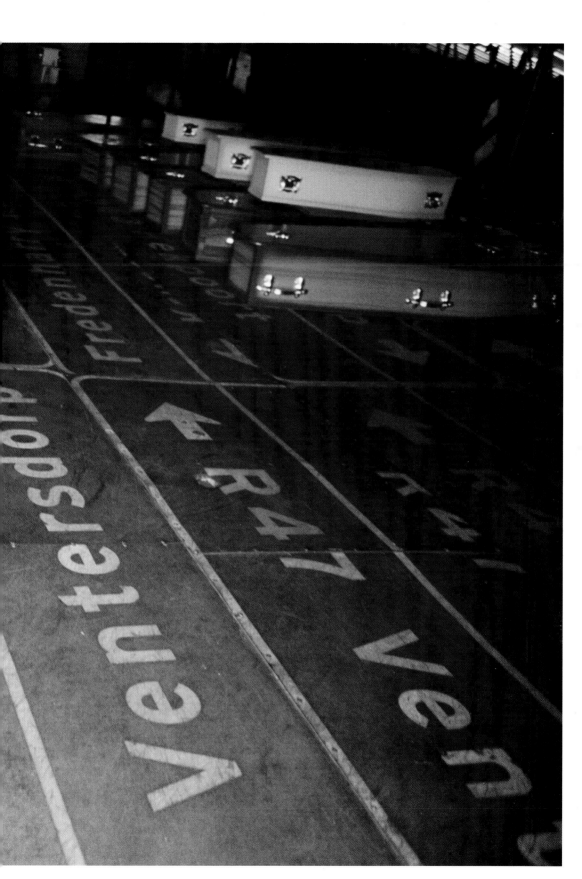

INTRODUCTION

The fastest-growing epidemic in the world

Why does HIV/AIDS have Southern Africa by the throat?

Responses to the epidemic

The first AIDS cases in South Africa were reported in 1983. At the time, few could have imagined the loss of life and the human suffering that we face today. At first the epidemic had its greatest impact among minority groups – intravenous drug users, prostitutes and gay men. This allowed those who did not belong to these 'high risk groups' to imagine that they were immune from infection. If you weren't a prostitute, didn't do drugs, and were straight you thought you were not at risk. Understanding of AIDS was strongly influenced by moral judgements. Minorities on the margins of

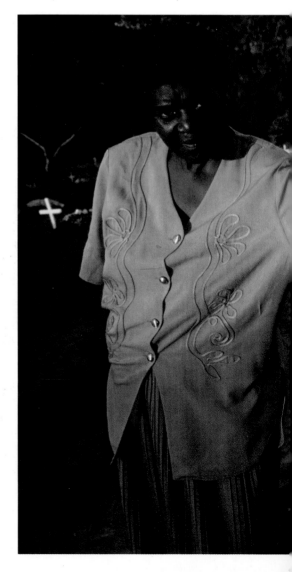

Community worker in Clermont, Durban, where every week graves are dug for the many youth who are dying of AIDS

society were often blamed for the spread of the disease. Those who were infected were believed to be the victims of their own immoral or antisocial behaviour. And these perceptions added to the stigma attached to AIDS.

Warning lights started to flash in the mid-1980s, when several migrant workers tested HIV positive. By 1989 it was clear that the AIDS epidemic in the Southern African region was mainly heterosexually transmitted. But the spread of the disease did not put an end to the practice of blaming.

Unsurprisingly in apartheid South Africa, racial and political attitudes strongly influenced people's attitudes to AIDS. Some blacks argued that whites had deliberately spread the disease and that the promotion of condom use was a racist device to curb the growth of the African population. These ideas were encapsulated in a popular expression at the time: that AIDS stood for 'American Invention to Destroy Sex'.[1] Some whites saw AIDS as a disease that was mainly restricted to black people, while a deeply racist fringe celebrated its destructive impact on the African population.

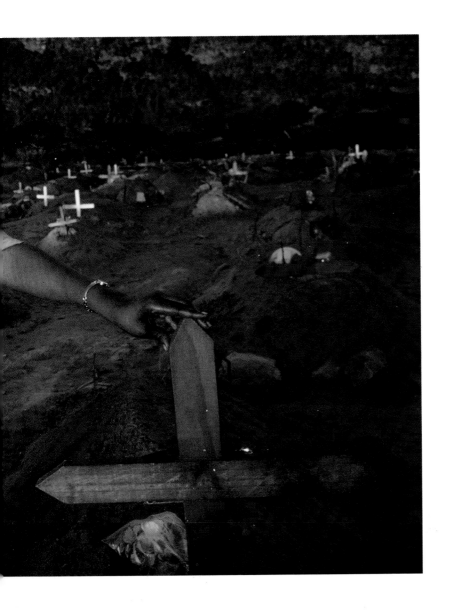

THE FASTEST-GROWING EPIDEMIC IN THE WORLD

While these debates rumbled on, the region faced the largest and fastest-growing epidemic in the world. South Africa is said to have more people living with HIV (Human Immuno-Deficiency Virus) than any other country. By 2005, most Africans will die before they reach their 48th birthday.[2] The World Health Organisation (WHO) estimates that by 2010 life expectancy in South Africa will be 43 years, seventeen years less than it would have been before the epidemic. In Harare, the Zimbabwean capital, 340 people die every day, 240 of them from AIDS-related illnesses. According to the curator of cemeteries for Harare, there is a government campaign to encourage cremation because 'We are running out of space in the graveyards. At the moment in our two open cemeteries [the other five are full] we have two burials per hour, every hour, between 10 am and 3 pm, seven days a week.'[3]

Zimbabwe could easily be seen as a model of South Africa's future. Already, cemeteries in Johannesburg have widened their entrances to allow buses carrying mourners to enter side by side, and loved ones are buried in cardboard coffins.

As the tables below show, rates of infection have rocketed over a comparatively short period and the region faces profound social upheaval and terrible loss of life.

The epidemic is also having a devastating impact on the youngest members of society. One-third of infants born to HIV-positive mothers are infected and very few will live beyond the age of 6. A study conducted at the perinatal clinic at the Chris Hani Baragwanath Hospital in Soweto found that 'one in three babies born to mothers diagnosed HIV-positive dies within twelve months, compared to one in fifty-nine babies born to HIV-negative mothers'.[4]

The emotional cost and economic burden to families and communities are vast. Parents and grandparents bury children and die prematurely themselves. Children and old people battle to keep their families together in the absence of parents. Children as young as five collect water and firewood, harvest crops and prepare food. They leave school early to support siblings, dying parents and grandparents.[5] They care for sick and dying relations with little or no support, and do not qualify for child-support grants because they are children themselves.

Estimated HIV infection in 2000, aged 15 – 49

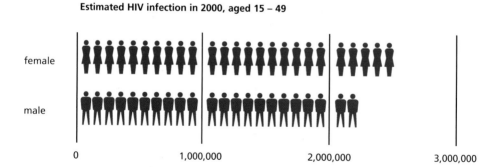

The number of deaths is overwhelming. As leading South African scientist Professor Malegapuru Makgoba has said, 'If we had been involved in a major war, that would be the only other thing that could explain the high numbers of young men and women who are dying in our country.'[6]

It is important to consider the emotional impact of the epidemic on people's daily lives. Vusi Ngema, who never goes out except to the clinic because people think he looks like someone with AIDS, voices his frustration:

My life has no hope. Why doesn't the Lord just take me? I will feel better if I am dead. My main worry is that I am a burden to my family. Most of the time I feel so stressed I don't talk to anyone. I just want to be left alone. I have headaches and a stiff neck and stiff shoulders. It is as if I am carrying something very heavy. There is nothing that I do. I get washed. My mother brings me my breakfast porridge in bed. Usually, I only get up at around 1 pm. Then I sit and listen to the radio for a while. After I am tired of sitting, I go and lie down again.[7]

In 2000, it was estimated that there were 2.5 million HIV-positive women aged 15 to 49, and 2.2 million HIV-positive men aged 15 to 49 in South Africa.

Recent projections of HIV-infected individuals indicate that these figures could reach 7.5 million by 2010. This represents a fifth of the population.

In the period 2000 to 2010 between four and seven million South Africans may die of AIDS-related illnesses. The number of AIDS deaths will be much larger than the number of those due to any other single cause. It will be almost double the number of deaths from all other causes combined over that period.[8]

It is estimated that there are an average of 1500 new infections and 600 AIDS-related deaths every day.

Estimated increase in HIV infections 2000 – 2010

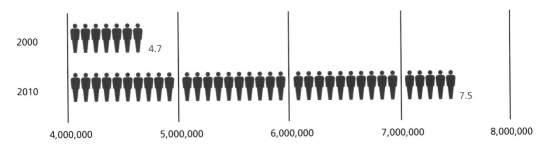

WHY DOES HIV/AIDS HAVE SOUTHERN AFRICA BY THE THROAT?

Poverty and disease are widespread in Southern Africa and are major factors in the rapid spread of HIV and subsequent opportunistic infections.[9] The disease mainly affects poor households in the region because breadwinners are ill or dying. The loss of income due to illness and medical and funeral expenses can be a devastating blow to an already desperate family. It can also pitch families that were just able to make ends meet into poverty. 'The financial impacts of HIV/AIDS on households are as much as 30% more than [those incurred by] deaths from other causes.'[10] This is because the cost of treating AIDS-related illnesses is high, and many families have experienced a loss of income due to prolonged ill health.

Because professional health services are limited, the burden of care rests with the family, particularly the women. *Stokvels* (informal credit associations) and burial societies are among the few sources of support in poor communities but their resources are stretched to breaking point by the rising death rate.

HIV is making existing social problems worse. Southern Africa's long history of forced population migration has torn families apart by separating mothers and fathers from each other and from their children. The region has also been racked by intense social conflict and wars. This has contributed to the spread of the virus, because war results in destabilisation, the breakdown of families, rape, prostitution and the constant movement of soldiers across borders. In South Africa, massive social inequalities, where 'unparalleled impoverishment exists side by side with unimagined accumulations of wealth', further aggravate the situation.[11]

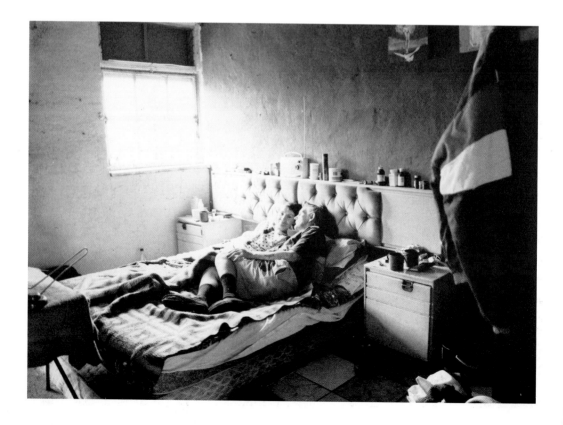

The system of migrant labour was characterised by poor working conditions, occupational health risks, and overcrowded and unhygienic accommodation. This resulted in poor nutritional status and lowered immunity, which made people susceptible to many diseases including tuberculosis (TB). The separation of families, economic vulnerability and bleak living conditions created an environment in which sexually transmitted infections (STIs) were commonplace. It is now well known that the presence of TB and STIs is associated with the rapid spread of HIV/AIDS because these diseases compromise immunity. Open genital ulcers from STIs also provide fertile ground for the transmission of the virus. Prof. Makgoba comments, 'We have multiple small epidemics which are coalescing – a result of migrancy and the huge burden of STIs.'[12]

Deep-seated gender inequalities have also contributed to the rapid spread of HIV/AIDS.

Violence against women is a crucial factor in this. South Africa has the highest level of rape of any country not in a state of war. Many women are infected through rape and are unable to get the drugs they need to help prevent HIV infection. Sexual violence in the home is widespread. It is estimated that one woman in six is in an abusive relationship. For example, studies have shown that up to 80% of women in rural areas have experienced domestic violence. This is a huge problem because it is not possible to negotiate safer-sex practices in abusive relationships.

(Left) The Ark Christian Ministries shelter in Durban is a homeless and indigent shelter and care centre. According to the shelter's AIDS co-ordinator, 400 of the 900 residents are HIV positive.

(Right) Malinkana Chokwe (13) cooks porridge for her six brothers and sisters

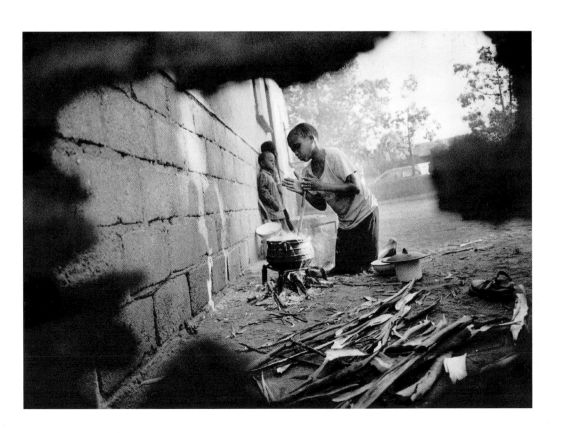

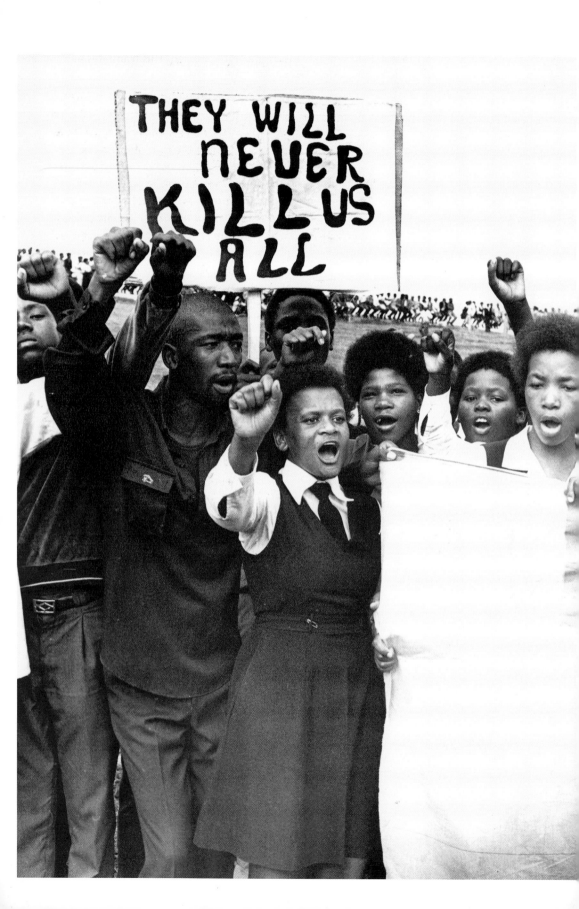

RESPONSES TO THE EPIDEMIC

The combined efforts of government, Non-Governmental Organisations (NGOs), the private sector, churches and communities have not slowed down the rate of infection. However, HIV/AIDS is not an inevitable outcome of poverty. Countries with similar social circumstances, such as Uganda and Senegal, have not seen such a rapid spread of the epidemic. This means that the spread of the disease is also influenced by personal choices, political responses and cultural factors. Why has South Africa failed to slow down the spread of the disease?

The HIV/AIDS epidemic arrived at a time when the turbulent process of political transition dominated the thinking of most leaders. In the face of imminent political disaster, the longer-term danger posed by the epidemic seemed less significant.

Economic constraints, such as the competition for limited government resources by sectors like education, housing and health, meant that the government's response was inadequate at best. By 1992/93 the AIDS budget still fell far short of the WHO's recommended R143 million a year. In five years it had grown from R1 million to just R22 million per year.[13]

There is a sharp division between the rich and the poor in South Africa. Those who are most in need receive the least treatment and care. In a population of 43 million people, only 19% are on medical aid. Medical aid schemes have recently expanded their AIDS-management programmes but this sector only caters for the rich. Of an estimated 4.7 million infected people, only about 20 000 to 30 000 are receiving HIV treatment in the private health sector. It is very difficult for people who are HIV positive to obtain medicines for opportunistic infections from public health facilities.

The struggle against apartheid: protesters at a funeral, 1984

One reason for the slow response to the disease is social stigma. The virus carries the stigma of being primarily sexually transmitted. Other STIs are now curable. AIDS is not. With AIDS, pleasure and death run hand in hand. The virus is complex and it takes a long time for symptoms to show. The epidemic is distinctive in that it is unseen – people can look and feel healthy for years while carrying the virus. This invisibility of infection impedes AIDS education programmes. If infected people look and feel healthy it is possible to deny the existence of the disease. The long gap between infection and death has enabled the government to ignore the looming crisis.

Initial research has been largely confined to the biomedical sciences. Public health intervention strategies have been informed by this narrow scientific reasoning, which sees individual sexual behaviour as the major cause of transmission and therefore the focus of change. But AIDS is a profoundly social epidemic, so it is hardly surprising that interventions targeting individual behaviour have proved to be inadequate.

Few can question the influence of gender, poverty, violence and cultural norms on the spread of the disease. However, there is no single explanation for the HIV/AIDS epidemic in South Africa. A unique combination of factors influences the pattern and profile of the epidemic. The mix of poverty, violence, rapid political change, migrancy and sexual networks has created an environment in which the disease is spreading at an unprecedented rate.

Sex, power and risk lie at the heart of understanding HIV/AIDS in contemporary South Africa. Thus, making sense of sexuality and gender is a central concern of this book. Men drive the HIV/AIDS epidemic, and gender inequality, violence and sexual coercion all contribute to the spread of the disease. Masculinity takes many different forms and in South Africa these can be extreme, ranging from gangster to father and caregiver. So in order to comprehend and curb the epidemic we need to understand men's sexual behaviour.

A distinctive feature of the South African epidemic is the number of children infected with HIV/AIDS. This is not simply due to transmission at birth. Young people often experience sex early in life and in coercive circumstances and this increases the risk of infection. The number of AIDS orphans is also alarmingly high. Children are obliged

'I speak of the gap between rich and poor, not as an observer or as a commentator, but with intimate personal knowledge. I am an African. I am living with AIDS. I therefore count as one among the forbidding statistics of AIDS in Africa. Amid the poverty of Africa, I stand before you because I am able to purchase health and vigour. I am here because I can afford to pay for life itself.'[14]
– Mr Justice Edwin Cameron, International AIDS Conference, Durban, 2000

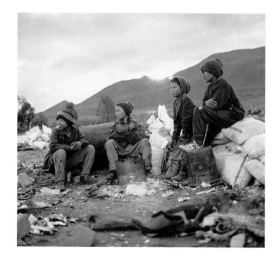

to assume adult responsibilities and the burden of care falls on elderly people and the government.

It is vital to have a historical and cultural perspective on HIV/AIDS if we are to understand the course of the epidemic in Southern Africa. Specific historical features like migrant labour, urbanisation and the demise of generational authority have fuelled the spread of the disease. The vast disparities of wealth on the subcontinent exacerbate the impact of HIV/AIDS.

How people make sense of disease and illness also helps to explain their perceptions of transmission and treatment. Historically, marginal groups have been blamed for being the source or cause of the disease. Ironically, key organs of state control, such as the CIA or the South African security establishment under the apartheid regime, have also been the locus of blame. Some rural African communities see AIDS as a resurrection of old African diseases that have assumed a new virulence because of disrespect for culture. The exchange of fluids in sex is linked to strong cultural beliefs associated with well-being. Some of the symptoms of AIDS are closely associated with *isidliso* – a form of poisoning inflicted by witches.

Witchcraft is a popular explanation for the origins and symptoms of AIDS.

Earlier cultures are being reinvented in modern South Africa and traditional culture today bears little relation to culture 150 years ago. Virginity testing is an example of this. This book tries to plot the dynamic and evolving nature of tradition. Lessons from past epidemics show that social divisions and prejudices are exacerbated in moments of social transition. In this respect the HIV/AIDS epidemic has shown itself to be no different. One of the main challenges facing South Africans today is how to stop the spread of HIV/AIDS. Yet we don't have a full picture of the epidemic. One reason for this is the lack of adequate social research that could inform HIV/AIDS prevention and the separation between research and implementation. This could help to explain why public health campaigns have failed.

The key contribution of social science research on HIV/AIDS is to situate the individual in relation to his or her social, cultural and historical environment; in other words to locate 'AIDS in Context'. Through this book we aim to continue the conversations started at the conference, to impart existing research and to stimulate further inquiry.

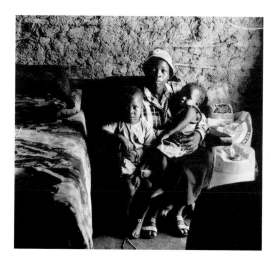

(Left) Children from Calvinia, Northern Cape, 2002
(Right) HIV-positive mother from KwaZulu-Natal with her two children

SEX AND POWER IN SOUTH AFRICA

Being a man in South Africa

Being a woman in South Africa

Being a child in South Africa

In sub-Saharan Africa, 55% of HIV-positive adults are women. In South Africa twice as many women between the ages of 15 and 24 are HIV positive than men in the same age group. And in South Africa as a whole twelve to thirteen women are currently infected for every ten men. How do we explain this? As we show in this chapter, biologically it is easier for women to contract the virus. But this only partly answers the question. In order to understand the pattern of HIV transmission in South Africa we need to understand how men and women interact socially and sexually.

Sex is social – whom we have sex with, how and where we have sex, our views about sexual morality and even the objects of our sexual desire are not necessarily individual choices. The environment in which we live influences the extent to which we are able to control these choices. Sex is also about power – who initiates sex, who makes the decisions, who decides whether or not to wear a condom. These decisions are contested because relationships between men and women are unequal. In order to make sense of the AIDS epidemic we need to look at the social context and power dynamics that inform sexual behaviour, and understand sexual relationships and gender inequalities between men, women and children.

Gender inequality interacts with other social factors, for example poverty, generation and race. One way that gender inequality is manifested is in the extent and nature of sexual violence. In South Africa sex is often the site of routine violence and brutalisation. In 1998, for example, a total of 54 310 sexual crimes were officially recorded, though the actual figure was much higher.[15] And it is impossible to negotiate safer-sex practices in a climate of violence and abuse.

Understanding sex and sexuality in their social context has direct implications for the development of HIV/AIDS prevention pro-grammes. So far these programmes have focused on changing individual sexual behaviour, and they have failed. For example, interventions have encouraged men to wear condoms and women to insist that they do. But this is often impossible. For some men and women, the exchange of fluids during sexual intercourse is linked to strong cultural beliefs about maintaining good health. And if condom use is culturally taboo, then a programme that promotes condoms is unlikely to succeed. For example, the Botswanan government's prevention campaign, run under the banner of 'ABC' (Abstain, Be Faithful and Condomise), had very little impact because it did not take into account cultural beliefs around fluid exchange.

There are sharp divisions between rich and poor in South Africa. Divisions also exist within and across different communities. Wealthy suburbs exist alongside poor ones. There are also clear divides between rich and poor within poor communities. In other words there are different levels of inequality. In this environment sex becomes something to be exchanged for material goods. For women who are desperate it is a way of survival. For others, it is a way of acquiring commodities. Transactional sex flourishes in this setting. It is often the only available currency. The transactions can take many forms, and in some communities extensive vocabularies have developed, for example to describe the status and value of boyfriends. Transactional sex should not be conflated with prostitution, though, which involves clear commercial exchanges between sex workers and clients. Transactional sex describes a range of sexual relationships in which there is a mutually agreed exchange of material goods for sexual services. It reflects the power relations between 'provider and recipient'.

In 1993 in South Africa, the richest 10% of the population received 47.3% of the income, whereas the poorest 40% of the people only had a 9.1% share. Land inequalities mean that 71% of the rural population – mainly black – lived on 14% of the land, while the balance of farmland was owned by 67 000 farmers, almost all white. The same situation obtains in Zimbabwe, although here the 'land reform' means that the major landowners are black cronies of the leadership. There are also regional inequalities: in 1998, per capita income in Mozambique was US$210, in Lesotho US$570 – compared to South Africa's US$3310.[16]

BEING A MAN IN SOUTH AFRICA

The global AIDS epidemic is driven by men. Men have more opportunity to contract and transmit HIV; men usually determine the circumstances of intercourse; and men often refuse to protect themselves and their partners.[17]

Ironically, men's greater social power places them in a position of vulnerability regarding HIV infection. Many of them are under social pressure to behave in a domineering and sexually aggressive way. 'For men, norms and expectations surrounding masculinity put them at risk.'[18] In addition, the norms of masculinity, which dictate that young men should be knowledgeable and experienced about sex, increase the risk, as such expectations prevent them from seeking information about safer sex. They may also be coerced into experimenting with unsafe sex to prove their manhood. Traditional notions of masculinity are strongly associated with risk-taking behaviour such as increased alco-

hol consumption, intravenous drug use, multiple sexual partners and violence. And these all contribute to HIV infection.

There is no single way of being a man. The roles that men play in society reflect different experiences of manhood – they are fathers, husbands, sons, boyfriends, and friends. Men constantly shift between these roles. Different communities have varying expectations of their men. For example, a church community may promote the values of sobriety, restraint, family responsibility and spiritual leadership, while a youth gang values bravado, prowess and violence. Being a man is also defined in relation to other men, women and children. For example, in a household a man may be expected to make all the important decisions, discipline the children and control the family resources.

Risk-taking behaviour, social norms and pressures and multiple roles all have an impact on male sexuality. In the context of risk-

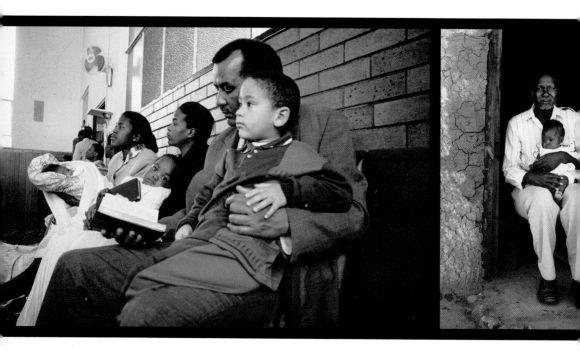

taking behaviour this may mean having
unsafe sex with multiple sexual partners. So
men's individual choices are influenced by
societal norms. The same set of expectations
can lead to a positive or negative outcome.
The idea of men being dominant and in control could spark violent behaviour but may
also include men assuming responsibility for
providing, protecting and caring for their
families.

Many of these themes were reflected in the
papers presented at the AIDS in Context
Conference. Most of the research was based
on specific case studies, for example male
youth in Owamboland in Namibia, students
in Zimbabwe or women living in deep rural
areas. However, certain themes and patterns
emerge from these case studies. Details may
differ but some aspects of masculinity are
common. What we present here is an
overview.

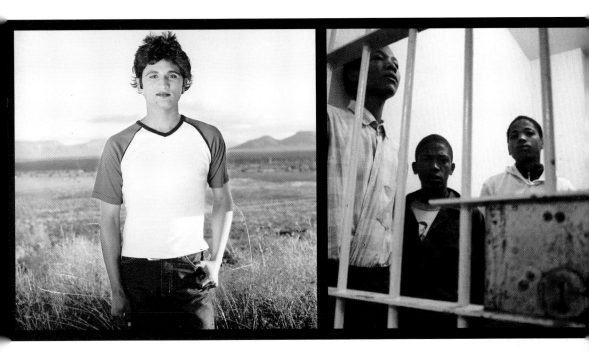

Achieving masculinity

Most studies show masculinity as rather fragile, provisional, something to be won and then defended, something under a constant threat of loss. [19]

How do men prove their manhood? A number of case studies undertaken in Southern Africa identify dominant behaviour in men. These include having multiple sexual partners, exercising control over women, coercive sex, violence between men, and the use of alcohol and drugs. Of course, not all men behave in this way. For example, some men place a high value on fatherhood and providing for their families. Different communities also have different ideas about what it means to be a man. Masculinity is achieved in a variety of ways and is often accompanied by unrealistic expectations and pressures.

Having multiple sexual partners
     Some men express their maleness by having sex with many different partners. There are numerous reasons for this. Some authors suggest that it could be a mark of virility, a product of uncontrollable male sexual urges. It is also explained through ideas about the traditional practice of polygamy. According to one researcher, the roots of promiscuity amongst Owambo youth living in the urban centres of Namibia are to be found in dispossession and poor economic prospects, and can be traced back to traditional norms of manhood in rural Owamboland. Traditionally, Namibian boys became men when they got married and owned land for agricultural purposes.

According to our tradition people have traditional houses. You are not the one to decide where you are going to stay, it's your parents. They have to look for land with good soil, for growing *mahangu*, for example. Before the house is built your father decides where it is going to be situated. He will tell you, 'my son, you are big enough, you are going to build your house here, your room must be here, your first wife's place

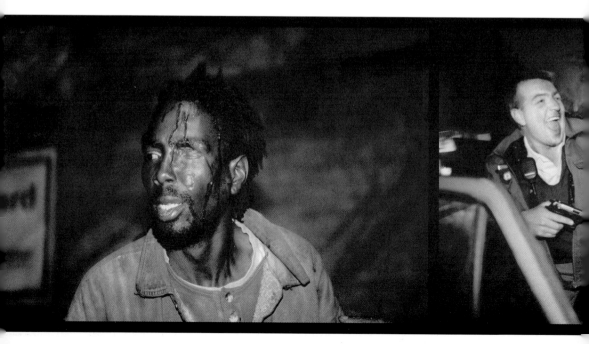

must be on this side.' This process means that you are being given a key.[20]

In an urban setting, Owambo boys also only 'become men' when they are economically independent and married. However, because of high levels of unemployment their economic prospects are very limited and they have had to find other ways of proving their manhood. One way is through having sex with many women. But while men have multiple partners, women are expected to be monogamous. As one Owambo youth put it: 'If you have many girlfriends then you are on top. You are a man ... if a girl has too many boyfriends then people start calling her names. They'll call her *oshikumbu*.'[21]

Men may react violently towards women who are not monogamous. A study conducted across several regions in South Africa found that 'boys believe that a way to sort a girl with several other sexual partners ... is to force sex or to "beat her" ... a girl who refuses [sex] and is believed to have another

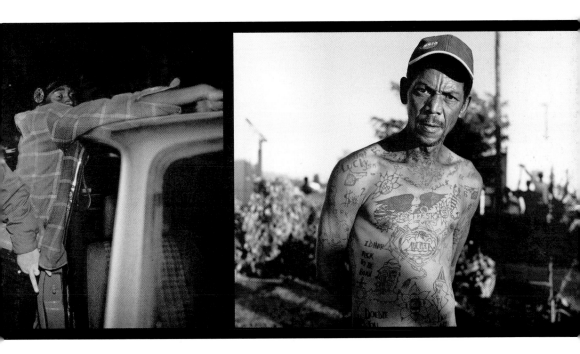

boyfriend will be beaten because "you cannot let her get away with it, she is using you and making you a chicken / a fool."' Some boys actually said 'ubufebe buqedwa yisibhakela', which literally means 'a punch puts an end to bitchiness' (a girl sleeping around).[22] A punch is mild compared to some of the punishments commonly meted out to girls suspected of having other partners. 'Some boys are fully prepared to sort out a girl whom they believe to be having other partners. A "steam-line" (istimela), commonly known as gang rape, is organised and carried out at the boyfriend's home to punish her for her actions.'[23]

The connection between violence, power and sex is perhaps most evident in South African prisons. Sexual transactions in prisons are controlled by gangs, which force some men to become 'wives' to more powerful prisoners. 'Sex in prisons is highly coercive in nature even when it falls short of direct rape.'[24] In the deprived environment of prison, sex may be exchanged for small privileges or simply used as a survival strat-egy. In prison, power is equivalent to manhood, so by raping another man the attacker seeks to 'validate his male dominance and superiority'.[25] Coercive sex in prisons is 'extremely pervasive'.

A warden at the Barberton prison sexually assaulted boys and gave them cigarettes or ten rand not to report him to the authorities. Gang members frequently raped newcomers as a form of initiation. At the holding cells in the Acornhoek police station, the entire 28 Gang had thigh sex with newcomers inside a shelter made from blankets.[26]

As this example shows, relationships based on violence are not limited to those between women and men, but also exist between men.

There are a number of reasons why men have multiple sexual partners. A contemporary study of youth in the Western Cape found that men believed that they could not survive physically or psychologically for an extended period without sex – a man need-

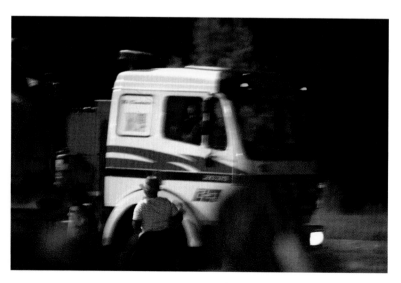

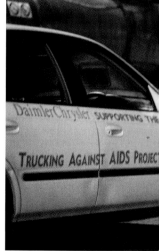

ed a back-up if his regular partner was not available. One young boy said, 'Hey man, there is this thing called AIDS, we should try to avoid this thing.'[27] But others said, 'No man, if AIDS means to stop having many partners then I will just contract it – you see.'[28]

Young boys from Limpopo Province also see male sexuality as uncontrollable:

When you're fifteen years old, your blood may start working and you will fail to control it. Even if your blood wants sex while you don't have anything [a sexual partner] it is no use to resist. What I am saying is that when you are fifteen your feelings can rise up and you will be ready to sleep with the girl. You cannot wait until you are 20 years old. It may be possible but it will be very difficult. Your blood rises and you go and look for a girl to drain this from your body. You can use a condom – you just need to drain something from your body.[29]

Sexual desire is seen as something that makes young men irrational. The man is

'Trucking against AIDS' trainers travel around South Africa visiting what they term 'hot spots' – truck stops and truck rest areas which are ideal sites for a thriving sex trade – and educate prostitutes and truck drivers about sexually transmitted diseases (STDs), particularly HIV/AIDS. As a profession truck drivers have one of the highest incidences in South Africa of HIV/AIDS, and the road freight industry estimates that three truckers a day die of AIDS-related diseases.

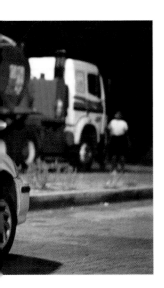

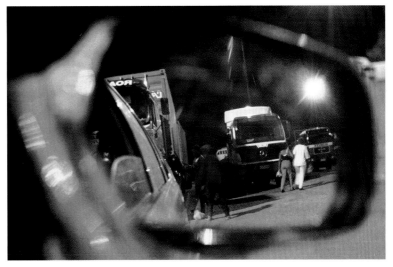

referred to as 'becoming confused', 'having feelings that affect his mind', and 'becoming slightly mad'. 'When a guy has sex, he becomes confused. He has a lot of feelings that affect his mind ... his voice changes and he seems to be whispering. His buttocks become stiff and he can start shivering.'[30] Even young men with steady girlfriends said that they fooled around with what they called 'roll-ons'. The word 'roll-on' refers to a stick of deodorant and is a metaphor for secret and hidden sexual partners. This has direct implications for HIV/AIDS interventions, as some young boys believe that condoms should only be used with the 'roll-ons' and not with their main partner.[31]

Young women and men also use cultural norms to explain why it is appropriate for African men to have many partners. In a study of student identities and AIDS in institutions of higher education in Southern Africa, women students interviewed spoke in a relatively detached way about what they construed as the 'cultural' and historical expectations for men to cheat. 'Guys have been cheating, you know our grandfathers, there are two families, there's the older wife and the younger wife. You know it's just a generation thing, so who are we now to change that thing?'[32]

Men in KwaZulu-Natal often use the image of the traditional 'polygamous patriarch' to suggest that multiple sexual partners are part of Zulu culture. As a young woman, said: 'They say it is their culture to have more than one girl. They say, "My grandfather had six wives, I want to be like him."'[33]

Using sex as a means of control

For many young men, coercion is part of sexual interaction. It is a means of asserting sexual control over women. A young boy in KwaZulu-Natal is quoted as saying:

When they are going to make sex, he asked, he said, 'Can we make sex?' ... but she said, 'no'... the way I think, maybe he asked her again, maybe she replied and they just made sex ... she didn't scream or do anything ... or tell him she doesn't want it ... to her, no is yes.[34]

The following poem was written by a homeless man living in Johannesburg:

I never gave her a smile
By James Moleleki

I met a beautiful woman recently
But I never gave her a smile
Because the vision of HIV/Aids was next to me
I was scared to get the virus.
Yes I never gave her a smile

Because the challenge was on me
The feeling was moving around my body
But I told myself I must not be positive
Because I didn't want to find myself in danger
Yes I never give her a smile

Because the idea of HIV/Aids was next to me
I turn down an invitation to one luxury hotel
To meet the cruel killer HIV/Aids
Yes I never gave her a smile [35]

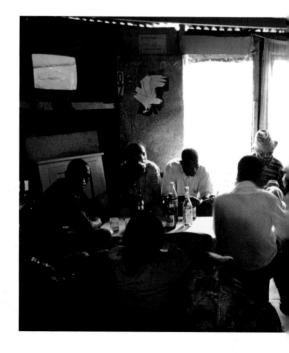

Some boys appear to identify unquestioned authority and control over women as a key feature of masculinity, and 'see themselves as having undisputed power over their girl-friends, that is, they feel they have control over them'.[36] Women are seen as the property of their boyfriends. Like any other personal property, they are bought, owned, defended and controlled, and men have exclusive rights to sexual intercourse with their girlfriends. In order to compete for women, men also need to be financially independent.[37]

However, control is not limited to sex. In a study on sexual health and violence among township youth in the Eastern Cape, boys as young as 12 and 14 said they felt the need to demonstrate control over their girlfriends.[38] This included telling them whom they could talk to, controlling their movements and slapping them when they were disobedient. The roots of this behaviour can be seen in women's position in society. 'We have found that women are drilled to be submissive to men, as they

Men drinking in a shebeen, Khayelitsha, a township outside Cape Town

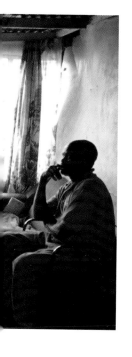

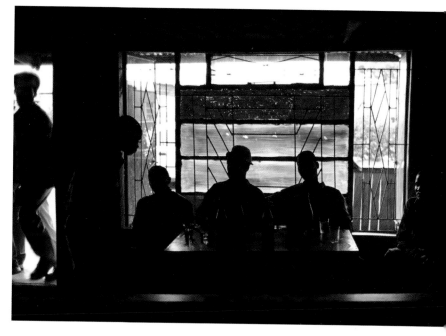

should be well-mannered. This translates as "they should know how to talk to a man." All the time they strive to please men, not only in the wider community but in their relationships as well.'[39]

Violence is a common expression of dominance and control over women. As a young man living in Windhoek explained, 'you beat her because you are the man. She must understand that I am the man. I am the boss.'[40]

Research into cultural beliefs and HIV/AIDS showed that both men and women believe that male sexuality is determined by biology – men have sexual urges that lead to inevitable behaviour patterns. There are two main aspects to this: firstly, the need to have many sexual partners, and secondly, the right to use force or violence. Young men and women believe that a man has a right, or even a duty, to force himself on a woman who displays reluctance and shyness.[41]

Similarly, respondents in a study of teenage masculinity did not see that forcing a girl to have sex was rape. Rape is an attack by a stranger. The study focused on the language teenagers use to talk about sex. Drama and role-plays indicated that the boys did not recognise that saying 'no' was an option for girls – they believed that girls should not have any say in the matter at all. Again, they used biology (the male sexual urge) to justify men having sex on demand. The following is quoted from a discussion after a role-play:

Girl: Why do you keep on persuading her?

Boy: I have to satisfy my needs.[42]

Ideas about men's biological needs featured prominently in a recent study conducted in KwaZulu-Natal primary schools, which showed that

many men subscribed to the idea that they have a boundless sex drive that is insatiable. Thus they must have multiple sexual partners … some men have been heard to say that women have weaker sexual organs, while they have strong and energetic organs, thus women must have limited sexual activity to preserve themselves.[43]

In a social setting where they are expected to be providers, men see themselves as failures if they can't fulfil this role. A long-term study of suicide in the Lowveld found that failure to provide for their families was a strong factor in male suicide.[44] Failure to provide can also make men aggressive and suspicious of their partners. A lack of authority in one situation, for example work, may result in men seeking to assert power in another, for example the household. This is the context for a lot of domestic violence.

Violence as a means of asserting power is seen not only in relationships between women and men but also in men's relationships with each other. A certain level of violence is even expected of young men. Public displays of violence allow young men to be seen as strong and heroic and to show off to girls. Men also feel pressured by peers to behave in this way.[45]

Violence and alcohol often go hand in hand. Amongst Owambo youth, drinking is very much part of being a man. 'If a guy does not drink he will never be accepted by his friends. They will call him a *moffie* [gay]. Life's no fun without alcohol … otherwise [i.e. if you do not drink] you are a useless guy.'[46] Heavy drinking and violent fights appear to be characteristic of male behaviour. A study of students at tertiary institutions in Botswana and Zimbabwe noted that 'real men behave badly': they get drunk and have sex with prostitutes.[47] The link between alcohol and forced sex has been identified in other research.[48] The boys interviewed in one study of teenage masculinity claimed

that forced sex was more likely to be perpe-
trated by boys who didn't have many girls
and who were drunk.

Achieving masculinity is about commanding
authority. Perhaps nowhere is this better
demonstrated than in Niehaus's study of
male sexuality on a mine compound. In this
instance masculine authority was the overriding factor. Niehaus noted that even when
female sexual partners were available in
nearby towns, men often chose to have relationships with other men. These relationships allowed older (more senior) men to
demonstrate their authority, and the 'comforts of home' provided by the young men
in the form of cooking, cleaning and sexual
services outweighed the sexual possibilities
of prostitutes or townswomen.[49]

Traditional male authority was undermined
by colonial authority and apartheid rule. For
many men the exercise of authority and control was restricted to the home. In post-
apartheid South Africa women's rights are
promoted and men's authority has been further undermined. A bit of dialogue from a
recent documentary about two men who
want to get married sums this up very well:

Is it okay if two men want to marry?

If men want to marry it's fine. A wife can change
into a man in your house. You may have to
cook, although you are a man. Now that this
rotten government gives women rights, you
can't solve your problems at home, because your
wife will run to the government. I'd rather be
with a man.[50]

The ways in which men achieve masculinity
have a direct bearing on the spread of STIs,
including HIV/AIDS. Understanding men's
attitudes towards condom use, safer-sex
options, trust, intimacy and responsibility
will help us to make sense of patterns of HIV
infection in South Africa.

Myths and prejudices about condoms

Young people are unlikely to perceive themselves as being at risk of contracting a
potentially fatal disease. Youth is seen as 'a
time of play, adventure and having fun
before the responsibilities of adult life pre-
vail'.[51] Youthfulness is closely linked with
experimentation and risk. As a schoolboy
from Bushbuckridge said, 'It is good to start
[having sex] at sixteen years because you will
have time to *jol* [have fun] before marriage.
And that will mean that you will remain
faithful in your marriage, because you have
had enough *jolling*.'[52]

In focus group discussions, playful relationships were contrasted with 'true love' relationships in respect of responsibility and
expectation. Condom use and contraception
were generally associated with the responsibilities of commitment and marriage. As one
young man put it, 'We will talk when we are
married so we won't discuss.'[53]

Youthful irresponsibility cuts across all sectors of society, rich and poor, black and
white. A study of university students found
that youth and casual sexual relationships
went together.

What about casual sex? … Especially in our age
group, I think it's the norm. I think that anyone
can go into a nightclub, pick somebody up and
go home and have sex. If that's what you want,
if that's your aim, it's no problem … It's very easy
… I know a lot of people who are doing that, it
happens, it happens often … A lot of people
shut up about it too, especially women, who
get labelled.[54]

However, although youthful irresponsibility
is given as one reason why condoms are not
used, there are many others. For some
teenagers, condoms have a stigma. Condom
use challenges the image of the healthy 'up-
and-coming man'. As one young man

reflected, 'I know you cannot see HIV but you look at her and you think "it is not there."'[55]

Both women and men say that using condoms reduces the pleasure of sex, and jokes about 'eating sweets with the wrapper on' and 'wearing a raincoat in the sun' demonstrate this. One study found that both men and women preferred 'flesh-to-flesh' (unprotected) sex for feeling. As one interviewee said, 'They tell you you won't feel anything of what you are doing if you are using plastic.' A female interviewee said, 'They say you don't fully enjoy sex. People want to feel the sperms when a man is ejaculating.'[56]

When men spend money on women there is an expectation that they can demand 'flesh-to-flesh' sex. The more they spend, the greater the expectation. As one interviewee said, 'He has been spending a lot of money so he will go for it, flesh to flesh.'[57]

Condoms are also seen as an awkward interruption in the 'heat of the moment'. The perception is that men lose control during sex, making condom use a secondary consideration. Condoms are about rationality, whereas sex is about passion and desire. 'When a man produces sperm (during sex), he becomes a little mad. You will see that he sweats a lot and the penis becomes erect, but he becomes strong. He feels like he is in heaven.'[58]

In a study of sexual meaning among youth in Limpopo Province, men spoke about diminished responsibility at the height of sexual passion. 'There is no time to speak. There is no time for discussion: you have to act quick.'[59]

Some women expressed similar sentiments:

I think, because I know from experience, that when you're still in a clothed state, the first

thing that's in your head is safety, etc. but the moment the kitters come off, I mean, your head sort of goes with them … Ja … And you accuse someone, 'oh, you silly girl', but I'm sorry, it's a different story when you're in that situation … Especially if you've had a few drinks … Your concerns go out the window …[60]

Sex is a natural enjoyable experience and condoms are seen as an unnatural intrusion on this. Some people didn't want to use condoms because they interfered with the sexual act. The future threat of AIDS was seen as less important than the immediate enjoyment of sex. A guidance teacher describes a conversation overheard at her school:

There's one class, they do talk about AIDS … a few of them they didn't really like the idea of using condoms because they said it's not natural, you know, and things like that, but for their safety they understand that they should. They don't agree with the idea of using condoms.[61]

If condoms are seen as unnatural, masturbation is even more taboo. Safer-sex programmes aimed at youth emphasise masturbation (and mutual masturbation) as an opportunity to experiment with sexuality. But views on masturbation are very clear. 'It plays with and confuses your mind … because you are trying to get that feeling and you are not there touching with a woman … you are just on your own.'[62]

One young man suggested that sex with a condom was like masturbation. He felt that sex must involve the exchange of fluids. There was a perception that failure to release bodily fluids during sex could lead to ill health. Bad skin is seen as a sign of this.[63] The importance of exchanging fluids is illustrated in this anecdote from a mineworker who only wore a condom when masturbating.[64] He said he was afraid of drawing in air. Had he been having sex with a partner, the exchange of fluids would have involved them both. In this instance he was afraid of being depleted and getting ill.

Interviews with male prisoners showed that they also see the lack of fluid exchange in non-penetrative sex as unhealthy.

Because the prisoners take male wives there will be a lot of disease. When men have sex between the thighs and ejaculate, their penises will suck air and they will grow lean. It is like masturbation.[65]

Those who think their lives will end in jail do that [have male–male sex]. But if you are a thinking man you won't. It is not good. When you have sex with a boy your penis will suck air into your body and there will be dirt in your lungs. After three years of doing that you will be infertile.[66]

Condoms have also become stigmatised because of the connotations of disease associated with them. People assume that if you want to use a condom you're sick. Wanting to use a condom is also seen as a lack of trust between partners. This is a very important part of negotiating condom use. If you love and trust someone, then why should you use a condom? Partners are often asked to express their love and trust by having unprotected sex. It can also be used to maintain a relationship or to prove that a marriage is monogamous.

A paper on how discourses of gender and sexuality affect safe-sex behaviour shows that 'love' is used to manipulate people into having unprotected sex. The assumption here is that relationships are monogamous, although this is often not the case. In sexual networks men often use condoms with their secondary partners but not with their main partners. Condom use has come to symbolise the status of the relationship.[67] Research in Hillbrow, Johannesburg, shows that sex workers use condoms with their clients but not at home because they believe that they can be infected by sex work but not by their regular partners.[68]

Limited knowledge of condoms and lack of access can also inhibit their use. Young people believe that obtaining condoms in public places such as clinics implies that they are sexually active, which many of them don't want to admit openly. The situation is made worse when nurses and clinic staff are hostile. 'The problem is that the nurses at the clinic are very unkind. Sometimes they even refuse to supply us with condoms ... they say we are troublesome. They think that we are not serious if we want condoms.'[69]

In the Durban area, at the heart of the AIDS epidemic in South Africa, young people also complained of the difficulty in getting condoms in clinics. 'When we go to the clinic they chase us away, saying we are too young ... They say you are wasting the condoms.'[70]

Even when condoms are available, men and women don't always know how to use them. Basic knowledge of condom use is limited and abstract. Some people had never seen a condom and many had never used one. Fears were also expressed about condoms, one of which was that they could 'slip off a man's penis during sex and get stuck inside the woman'.[71]

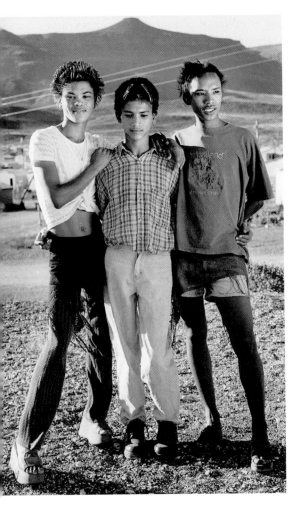

Cross-dressers from the small rural
town of Calvinia, Northern Cape

Male–male sexuality

Male–male sex is very pervasive in South
Africa. 'In the labour compounds and in
prisons male–male sex is not a practice of
peripheral others. It is part of the daily
encounters of ordinary masculine men.'[72]

Where this involves anal sex, the implications for the pattern of HIV transmission are
significant. Research has shown that HIV
transmission through unprotected anal
intercourse is much higher that unprotected
vaginal intercourse.[73] There is also a high
level of secrecy about male–male sex, and
the female sexual partners of men who practise it are often unaware of it. So this is
another pathway of HIV transmission that is
unspoken and under-researched.

HIV infection rates in the gay community are
also unknown. National statistics are drawn
primarily from antenatal clinics, which, by
definition, exclude gay men. In the initial
phase of the epidemic, the focus of attention was on homosexuality. However, with
the recognition that HIV is transmitted primarily through heterosexual sex, the health

Extracts from
'We Mourn Simon Tseko Nkoli'

On the eve of 1998 World AIDS Day,
30 November 1998, South Africa lost a freedom fighter, leader and activist to HIV/AIDS.
Simon Tseko Nkoli, a founder and leader of
the lesbian and gay movement, had died.

Delmas Treason Trial
In 1984, Simon Tseko Nkoli joined 21 comrades in the Delmas Treason Trial. His co-
accused included UDF and ANC leaders
Terror Lekota, Popo Molefe, Tom Manthata,
Gcina Malindi, and Moss Chikane. These
comrades spent more than four years on
trial for their lives. Some were then
imprisoned.

risks to the gay community have been large-ly ignored and under-reported. Health education campaigns are not specifically directed at homosexuals. There have been few studies on sexual networks and patterns of transmission amongst gay men. Those that do exist are micro-studies, usually focusing on factors that enhance or inhibit safer-sex practices.

In the West, prevention campaigns amongst gay men have been successful, largely because of shared characteristics within the community. This makes social mobilisation and public health messaging much easier. However, there are sharp differences in gay communities in South Africa. Experiences of gay men in a remote rural community are in stark contrast to the urban gay scenes of Johannesburg and Cape Town.

In South Africa many men who engage in same-sex practices do not identify themselves as being gay. Gender inequalities are often evident in same-sex relationships, where men are identified as feminine (*skesana*) or masculine (*injonga*) partners. In this model the *injonga* is dominant, sexually penetrating the *skesana* and maintaining a male social status, in contrast to the effeminate role and status of his partner. The high levels of domestic violence amongst heterosexuals are also found in homosexual relationships. Recent research on violence and particularly gang rape directed at lesbians shows that lesbians are becoming vulnerable to HIV infection in South Africa.[74]

Gay men who have gone public about their HIV status have made a significant impact in raising awareness within gay communities. Simon Nkoli, well known as an anti-apartheid and gay activist, spent the latter part of his life raising awareness about HIV/AIDS, especially among gay men.

In sum, regardless of sexual orientation, manhood and sex are intertwined throughout many men's lives.

Young, single men view sex as a rite of passage and a means of self-exploration, establishing masculinity and building self-esteem … For some older men, sex is an expression of love and the means of sustaining their lineage; for others it is a means of expressing their virility.[75]

During their detention, Simon Nkoli faced another trial, which changed the face of lesbian and gay politics in Southern Africa – he came out as a gay man. During many months of debate and discussion with his comrades and lawyers, Simon convinced these senior UDF and ANC leaders that lesbian and gay people faced discrimination. He confronted and destroyed the myth that holds that it is un-African to be gay.

HIV/AIDS
Justice Edwin Cameron, then a human-rights activist and lawyer, warned that HIV/AIDS would become the new apartheid. As the epidemic attacked the gay communities of South Africa, in a time when the National Party government neglected gay men and black people in the HIV/AIDS epidemic, lesbian and gay communities and activists mobilised. Simon Nkoli lived with HIV/AIDS for more than twelve years. As with many people, he faced racial oppression, homophobia and, now, AIDS-phobia. But after many years, Simon took on another burden – deciding to live openly with HIV/AIDS. There are more than three million people in our country living with HIV/AIDS, and Simon was one of the very few who said: 'HIV is a virus – not a shame.'

Today we say 'rest in peace, Comrade Simon Tseko Nkoli.' In Africa, you have created an army to fight oppression and injustice. We will defend your legacy and the equality of all people with HIV/AIDS.[76]

BEING A WOMAN IN SOUTH AFRICA

For women, the norms that define acceptable behaviour, economic dependency and violence have been said to make them vulnerable to HIV.[77]

All social relationships are characterised by an unequal balance of power between men and women. In South Africa this balance is heavily weighted in favour of men. Men are better educated, earn more than women, wield more power in society and have greater social status. Since South Africa's transition to democracy in 1994, these inequalities have been challenged by the state and the legal system. In fact, South Africa now has the most progressive constitution in the world. Nowhere is this more apparent than in the clauses dealing with gender relations. In spite of this, gender discrimination, sexual violence and oppression of women are rife.

The Constitution guarantees equality on the basis of sex, gender and sexual orientation; principles enshrined in the Bill of Rights and supported by several other clauses in the Constitution. South Africa is also a signatory to the Convention on the Elimination of all Forms of Discrimination Against Women. We have in place a comprehensive 'national machinery' for gender equality. South Africa is at the forefront of the Southern African Development Community region in terms of women represented at national, provincial and local government. At national level 29.8% of members of parliament are women – a higher proportion than ever before in the history of the country. Internationally these figures put South Africa in the top 10% of countries in terms of more equitable gender representation in various tiers of government.

Yet despite these positive signs, violence against women is endemic, both in and out-

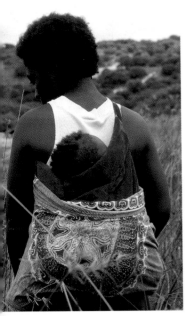

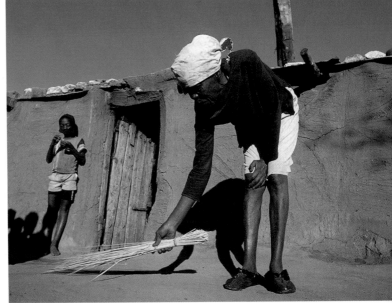

side the home. And rape statistics, while shocking, are regarded as underestimates owing to the high level of underreporting. Being a victim of a violent attack is almost an unremarkable part of being a woman in South Africa, and violence is a contributing factor to HIV transmission. For example, if a woman is forced into sex with an HIV-infected partner, her risk of infection is great. Also, women may hesitate to negotiate safer sex in an environment where they fear a violent response. Coercion is often a feature of sexual relationships from the outset. For example, in a study conducted in a rural area in the Eastern Cape, most women reported being coerced into early sexual activity against their wishes.[78]

Women bear the brunt of poverty and have the least access to resources. They have less access to education (for example, in 1995, 23% of African women aged 25 or more had no formal education, compared to 16% of

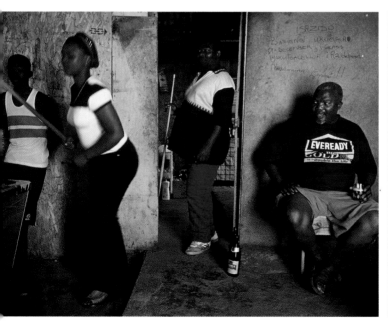
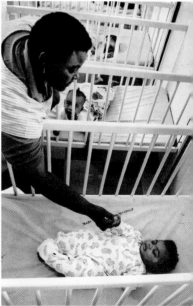

African men). Women earn less than their male counterparts (on average they earn between 72% and 85% of what men with similar education earn). They also bear the burden of unpaid labour, in particular childcare. And increasingly, they take responsibility for home care of the terminally ill. Young African women are the poorest, most economically marginalised and least educated sector of the South African population. This places them at the bottom of the health pile and renders them particularly vulnerable to HIV/AIDS.

There are also physical factors that make it easier for men to transmit HIV to women. 'Apart from solitary masturbation, vaginal intercourse is probably the most widely practised sexual act. In the absence of other factors, a man with HIV probably has a one-in-500 chance of passing the virus to his partner in a single act of unprotected vaginal intercourse. The odds of woman-to-man transmission in the same circumstances are about one in 1000.'[79]

STIs affect men and women differently. For instance, women are less likely to know they have an STI and also less likely to seek treatment for it, for cultural and economic reasons. Women's susceptibility is increased by other factors. Amongst these are genital mutilation, which can lead to bleeding during intercourse, and practices such as dry sex. A young woman is more at risk because of her immature genital tract, which has fewer layers of mucous membrane than that of an older woman. The amount of HIV (viral load) in semen is particularly high in the first few months after being infected. A man will transmit the virus to others during this time because he is more likely to have multiple partners and because viral load rises in seminal and not vaginal fluid.

What does it mean to be a woman in South Africa? How is 'womanhood' achieved and

negotiated? Research has revealed some of the patterns and trends of women's sexuality, experiences and behaviour, including harsh, often brutal experiences such as domestic violence and rape. But while studies highlight the negative and degrading aspects of women's lives in South Africa, women continue to play a pivotal and powerful role in their families and communities. Women are also challenging their circumstances and devising strategies to cope with and overcome adversity.

Some young girls have little opportunity to explore their sexuality in a context that is free of coercion or violence. And of course, HIV/AIDS adds an explosive and dangerous ingredient to this cocktail. In the past socially regulated sexual experimentation often involved forms of non-penetrative sex. Pregnancy and STIs were thus avoided.

One study focused on sexual debut among young women living in a deep rural area of the Eastern Cape. In this community there has been a recent change from non-penetrative sex to full intercourse at a young age. These young women are experiencing sex as something that happens to them rather than something they can initiate themselves. As many as 53% of the women interviewed who had had sex responded either 'unsure' or 'no' to the question 'do you like sex?'[80]

Sexual experimentation is controlled and discouraged among young women but encouraged among young men. Sexual initiation involves less obvious risks for men. Women, on the other hand, are in danger of getting pregnant, are more vulnerable to HIV infection, and are subject to violence and coercion. Throughout life women's sexuality is subject to strict social norms and expectations. One of these is the ideal of monogamous marriage; another is virginity. This is at odds with the expectation that men will have many sexual partners. The way women talk about love and romance reflects their personal aspirations as well as social pressures to conform. However, the reality of their sexual lives is often very different.

Female adolescents' notions of what to expect seem to be couched in ideal, romantic and unrealistic terms, and the reality seems to jolt them into suspension of all activities, for example, as one 35-year-old woman describes it, 'the first time was all very scary and ... I found the whole thing painful, it was not a very good experience; even now I don't know how I got used to it.'[81]

Unprotected sex as an expression of trust

Some women see marriage as a form of protection against HIV. Trust and intimacy are seen as an important part of marriage. One expression of trust is to have unprotected sex. This can be the case even when women know that their partners are cheating on them. 'I can't prevent him [from having other partners], but I trust him.'[82]

Female students in Botswana spoke about boys cheating on girls. They explained men's behaviour in cultural terms, saying that it was socially acceptable for men to have multiple sexual partners. When they discussed their own relationships, they expressed distress and resignation:

Rob: How do you feel about that [their boyfriends cheating on them]?
Lorato: Because the thing is, I can't say don't ... I have to get over the disappointment. I have to know that ... he's a man.
Wame: He's a man.
Lorato: Yes, so I have to face the reality that he's a man and he *will* cheat me.
Rob: So you expect him to cheat, do you?
Lorato: I *don't* expect him to cheat and he knows that I know that he can cheat ... I can only tell him you just cheat but don't ...
Wame: Don't let me know if he doesn't show you how are you going to know that he cheats

... You won't know so.
Lorato: Because when I say 'don't cheat' I'll sound so naïve.
Wame: Yeah.
Lorato: Because it happens.
Wame: It happens.
Masego: Every day.
Lorato: Our fathers cheat.
Wame: And the minute you hear about it you're going to be so ... you just shut things away because you think no one could do that to you because it's reality, it happens ...
Lorato: To everybody.
Rob: So you couldn't really imagine having a boyfriend who didn't cheat on you?
Wame: We'd love to.
Lorato: We'd love to. We'd love to.[83]

In respect of being monogamous, women, it appears, expect little of their men, while much is expected of them. However, despite the anticipation of male infidelity, they still see marriage as a safe haven. In fact, single women expressed envy of the 'safety' enjoyed by married women. Being married signifies a place of intimacy where condom use is not necessary. 'We are single, we need to use condoms, so those who are married, they are lucky.'[84]

These attitudes towards trust and intimacy also apply to long-term monogamous relationships. In this instance, the status of the relationship is measured by the willingness of the partners to take risks and practise unsafe sex. Unprotected intercourse is equated with love. But given the high level of cheating, marriage can be particularly dangerous. One woman who had only had one partner said: 'I was diagnosed through this child [pointing to her baby]. My child was very sick, then after the tests it turned out that the child is [HIV-] positive. I had that problem of where did I get it from because I always had one partner.'[85]

Sex as a resource

Some women have multiple sexual partners. This is often linked to their economic position. A study of transactional sex in KwaZulu-Natal uncovered different motivations for sex. Women in dire economic circumstances have sex so as to pay for basic necessities. Other women who are better off have sex to acquire a range of commodities. It seems that women who are unemployed and dependent on men for their economic survival tend to choose boyfriends as a way of making ends meet. A comment often made is that women *qoma* (choose a man), 'One for rent, one for food, and one for clothes.'[86]

Yet women still see themselves as having a choice. One young woman commented:

Sometimes she is loving someone who treats her badly, maybe he abuses her by hitting her or something. So she says, let me try another. But then she finds that he is also going to treat her badly. [Then] she will *qoma* another one, maybe she is looking for money. Others, they come from far, they want work, they end up having to *qoma* a lot of boyfriends because they can't find work. The men give them money for rent, food and clothes.[87]

For women in a slightly more secure economic position, boyfriends can be a source of extras or luxuries, such as designer clothing and stylish cell phones. Thembi, a young woman, felt it was important to be well dressed: 'You are nothing if you do not have fashion. I am scared to even leave the house; if you don't have something to wear, people laugh at you, they point at you and say, "look what she is wearing."'[88]

A young man wistfully reflected on the need to have an expensive cell phone:

With your Alcatel you will not get the *amaCherries* [women] most of the time. If you

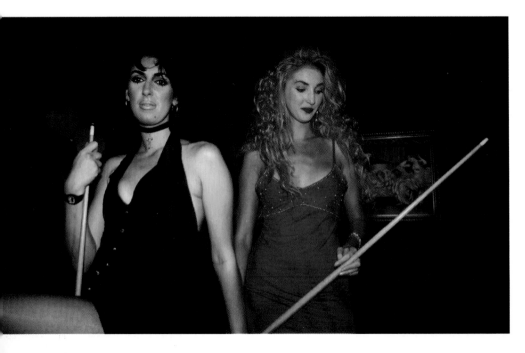

come with an Alcatel, it is a child's thing ... They want an expensive one, like a T28 or 6110. If you come with this little Nokia, they are going to respect you. If you come with the small Siemens, the C2, they respect you, they can see that you are the boss, you have money ...[89]

Sometimes the distinction between subsistence and consumerism is not all that clear. Clothes and new hairdos are used to attract boyfriends who will then provide basic necessities. This is illustrated in the following comments made to researchers Nonhlanhla and Philiswe by Thandi, a young woman living in an informal settlement:

Nonhlanhla: How many boyfriends do you have?
Thandi: Three.
Nonhlanhla: Why do you have three boyfriends?
Thandi: Because I have many needs.
Philiswe: What needs?
Thandi: To dress, I don't work, a cell phone ...

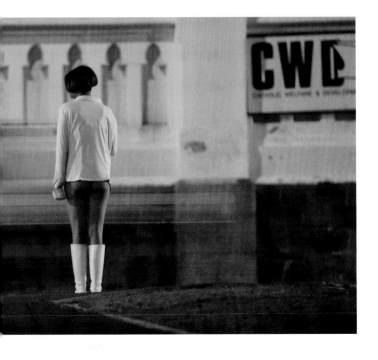

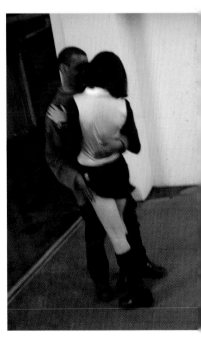

Mpume was tested for HIV only before starting sex work. She says that often her clients secretly break condoms. She is not currently on any other form of contraception but takes quinine tablets from the pharmacy, which she believes provide some protection.[93]

Doing my hair so that I am beautiful; for my boyfriends, they won't love an ugly person.

Nonhlanhla: What do they give you?

Thandi: One [gives] money … another Checkers groceries … another buys me clothes.

Nonhlanhla: Does your mother know where the groceries come from?

Thandi: She knows, she doesn't say anything because of the situation of hunger at home.

Nonhlanhla: Do other people know that you have many boyfriends?

Thandi: Yes, they know, my neighbours criticise me, but not in front of me, they gossip about me, they say that I am *isifebe*. But my friends, they understand the situation, they say nothing.

Nonhlanhla: Do you use condoms?

Thandi: With one, but two don't agree. These two say that they want *inyama enyameni, abafuni ukudla uswidi usephepheni* (flesh-to-flesh sex, they don't want to eat a sweet still in its wrapper) …

Nonhlanhla: What do your friends think about the future?

Thandi: They wish … like me one day, I wish to get the right person, who is going to love me and do everything for me and we marry.[90]

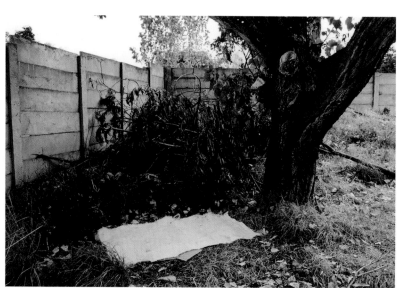

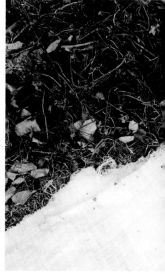

There are many kinds of transactional sex. Thandi and Thembi's stories are about the 'three Cs' – cars, cash and cell phones. They exchange sex for gifts. Another survival strategy is sex work – sex with multiple partners for money.

It is impossible to estimate the size and composition of the sex-worker population in South Africa. There are at least a dozen separate sectors of sex work – for example male, female, trans-gendered, urban, rural, commercial, casual, indoors, outdoors.[91] Sex workers come from a wide range of backgrounds. Education level and economic position vary. Many of them move in and out of the profession. In one study, a third of women polled had no employment other than sex work and half had had less than one year's experience in anything else. In a survey of 349 street sex workers in Durban, Cape Town and Johannesburg, a full 10% admitted to being under the age of 18.[92]

In a study of sex workers in Carletonville (the biggest gold-mining complex in the world), a number of themes emerged to explain sex workers' high levels of vulnera-

Condoms lie within arm's reach on the field beds of sex workers around the Far West Rand mineshafts of Carletonville. Women at high risk were the first people to be trained as peer educators and community-based condom distributors when Mothusimpilo – a community-based HIV/AIDS prevention programme – started in the area in 1998. Training enabled women to develop the skills to protect their health by requiring clients to use condoms. It also built social cohesiveness, enabling local sex workers to band together and collectively renegotiate the prevailing sexual culture.

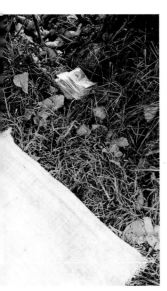

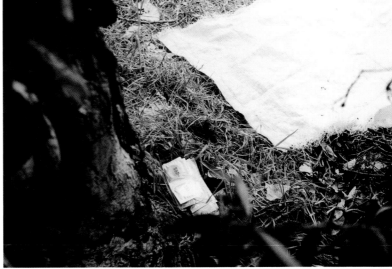

Toni's Story

Toni is a 22-year-old 'coloured' woman from Eshowe. She was sent to a reform school at the age of fifteen, after her father, a steelworker, sexually abused her. She estimates that 80% of the girls on the street have been abused by their fathers or stepfathers.

Toni demands her interview fee upfront, and directs me to an alley where she buys a crack rock, which she proceeds to smoke during the interview. She was recently hospitalised after overdosing on several massive hits of crack. She uses white pipes to come down at the end of the evening. She says crack 'makes her hot' and that it is a 'love drug'. She likes to use it when she 'needs TLC' and also to forget. She can spend as much as R1000 on crack a night.

She recollects one incident in which she was caught by two policemen with over R1000 of crack on her. They all smoked the drug together and she had sex with both cops. They let her go with the remaining rocks.

She worked as a bar lady and stripped at a seamen's club for two months before hitting the streets twelve months ago. She is not interested in working in an agency because 'I can't work for a boss. But some day I will be a madam.' The other sex workers are 'friends in need but not in deed', so she prefers to be alone. Her right eye is red and swollen during the interview – she says she got into a fight with another girl.

Her boyfriend of eight years dropped her last year, right before she hit the streets. She was in love with him. Her current 'sugar daddy' is interested in marrying her, but she is only interested in his money and has told him so. She is on the street the night of the interview because she had a fight with him.

She has one daughter, who is staying with her mother. She would really like to return home, despite her father's abuse. She just wants to lead a 'normal life'.[97]

bility to HIV infection. The majority of women had limited education and had lost contact with family support structures. A number of them had had previous experience of abusive and violent men. The most important factor, however, was the context of their working lives.[94] Miners were resistant to using condoms and financial hardship compelled women to go along with this. Unequal gender relations are particularly apparent in commercial sex work, where women are often powerless to insist on safer-sex practices. High levels of alcohol consumption amongst sex workers also reduce condom use.

Sex workers in Hillbrow in Johannesburg draw a distinction between safer-sex practices at work and at home. Most sex workers use condoms with their clients and many of them rely solely on condoms for contraception. 'They do so knowing that some men slip off the condom before entering and that government condoms frequently break.'[95] However, a number of sex workers do not practise safe sex in intimate relationships with boyfriends or husbands.

Women who are economically vulnerable may need to rely on sex as a resource. In a study of women living in a peri-urban area on the outskirts of Durban, it was found that over 90% of participants were dependent on men financially and that meeting their immediate needs for food and shelter overshadowed the long-term consequences of unsafe sex.[96] Sex can be used to secure basic needs such as food and clothing, or for luxury items. AIDS has changed the consequences of these transactions, and the patterns of HIV transmission reveal the sexual networking that takes place. Women's sexuality is informed by social expectation, personal aspirations and sexual customs.

Sexual customs and practices

Women's fertility is a sign of status in some communities. For example, women may be required to fall pregnant before marriage in order to prove they can have children. There is also a stigma attached to sterility among women. This creates tension between a woman's desire to have a child and the need to protect herself against HIV.

In a situation where a woman doesn't want to conceive, the responsibility for contraception usually rests with her. Many women use injectable or oral contraceptive methods, which allow them to assume control over their fertility. But obviously these methods do not help to prevent HIV and other STIs. One study suggested that the increased availability of injectable contraceptives has in fact led to an increase in sexual activity amongst young people, thereby inadvertently increasing the risk of HIV transmission.[98] Another study showed that condom use amongst women dropped dramatically when they used an injectable contraceptive method. In fact nearly half of former condom users had abandoned the use of condoms in favour of this method of contraception.[99]

Historically, women have had to take care of contraception. They are also expected to take primary responsibility for the prevention of STIs, in particular, through the use of condoms. 'Boys indicated that it is the responsibility of girls to seek protection; they also assumed that their partners were protected from conception.'[100]

Despite their general lack of power to make men wear condoms, the onus is also on women to practise safer sex. A woman's safety thus depends on her ability to negotiate the use of condoms with an often unwilling partner.

The fear of violence and the threat of abandonment can stop women from insisting on condom use. 'Even if I tell my partner, he will say, "Oh, you've got another man." He will hit me. If you don't give your man the right thing [condomless sex] he will leave you. Give him the right thing.'[101]

Another reason for women's lack of power to insist on condom use was the threat of economic loss. As one woman said: 'The problem is money, that is why we listen to our man every time, even when we say I don't want to use a condom, because of money, [and because] we have children. No one will support our children.'[102]

The use of contraception presupposes that women are sexually active. In some communities, retaining (and being able to prove) virginity is highly regarded. Virginity ensures that women's fertility is controlled through marriage. Ideally a woman will only bear her husband's children. The mid-1990s saw a resurgence of public virginity testing. This was done to prevent unwanted pre-marital pregnancy and was also a response to the HIV/AIDS epidemic. There are two interpretations of this practice. On one level it can be understood as a desperate measure, initiated by older women, to regain control over younger women's sexuality. It is an attempt to reinstate parental authority over adolescent girls by creating a moral code based on previous traditional practices. It is also an attempt by women to reassert some control over their sexuality and their bodies in the face of endemic violence and disease. Another viewpoint (held by organisations such as the Commission for Gender Equality and the Human Rights Commission) condemns it as a violation of women's right to privacy, bodily integrity and gender equality.

The arbitrary grading of girls into A, B and C-grade virgins has more to do with social perceptions than it does with biological testing. Once again the onus of HIV prevention rests with women. Men are not accorded any responsibility for preserving the virginity of young girls. It is the duty of the girls to maintain their 'purity'.

Another common practice is 'dry sex'. This is a high-risk activity because vaginal tears and abrasions increase the possibility of HIV

Virginity testing in KwaZulu-Natal, April 1998

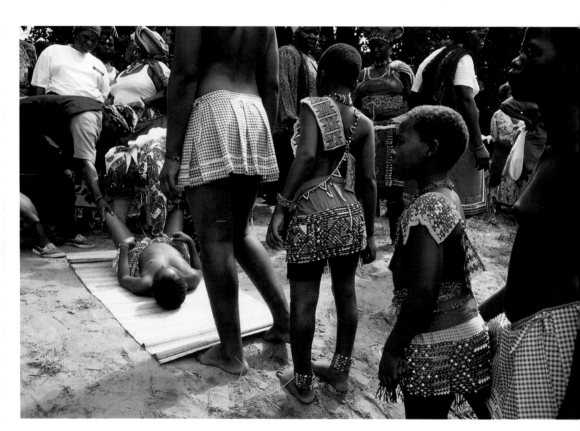

The ABCs of Virginity

Virginity testing refers to the practice of inspecting young girls to determine if they are sexually chaste. Some virginity testers grade girls according to a system derived from folk constructs rather than bio-medical knowledge.

Virginity is said to be evident if there is a visible 'white dot' somewhere deep in the vaginal canal. The hymen is described as a 'white, lacy barrier'. The barrier signifies that virginity is 'similar to the lace of a wedding veil'. Girls eager to pass their virginity test are said to resort to pushing toothpaste high up in the vagina to mimic the white lacy veil.

To achieve an 'A-grade' a girl has to meet a combination of criteria in which genital features are most important. The colour of the labia should be a very light pink, the vagina should be very small, the vagina should be dry and tight and the white, lacy veil should be clearly evident and intact. In addition, a girl's eyes should 'look innocent'. Her breasts and abdomen should be firm and taut and the muscles behind her knees tight and straight.

A 'B-grade' virgin is someone who may have had intercourse once or twice or 'may have been abused'. The labia of a B-grade virgin are a deeper

infection. Dry sex involves the use of sub-stances such as snuff, dry clothes and sponges as well as traditional herbs to tight-en and dry the vagina.

In other areas [of Tanzania] men prefer dry sex – little or no vaginal secretion – because, they say, their partners feel like virgins. 'A loose, wet vagi-na is a sign that a woman has had lots of sexual partners,' believes Peter, a 41-year-old civil ser-vant. To please their men, therefore, some women insert herbs, powders or pastes into their vaginas to make them dry and tight, although it makes intercourse difficult and unpleasant. 'When I am dry I get vaginal ruptures which get severe pains. I get pains for a week,' complains a woman from Dar es Salaam.[103]

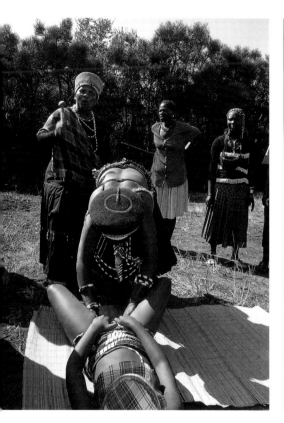

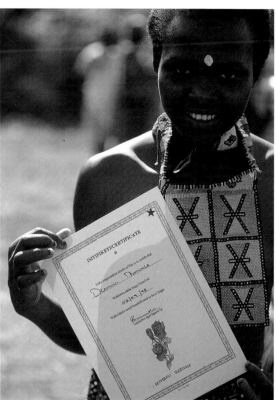

shade of pink, the vaginal opening is slightly big-ger, not so tight and the vaginal walls are slightly lubricated. The white dot and lacy veil are said to have 'been disturbed', although testers are reluc-tant to describe exactly what this looks like. A 'B-grade' girl's mother will be warned to watch her daughter closely, that someone has 'touched' her in an inappropriate way. She is declared a virgin and gets a certificate.

A vagina that is 'too wide and too wet', no evi-dence of a white dot or veil, eyes that 'know men', 'complicity in the sex act' or repeated abuse get a 'C-grade'. Most virginity testers say it is useless to do anything further for such girls as 'it is too late', 'nothing will change them'. A minority claim to counsel these girls about the dangers of sexually transmitted infections, AIDS and pregnancy, but at the testing events attended by the author there was little evidence of any kind of counselling.

A 'C-grade' is a mark of shame and disgrace. The girl's family may pay a fine. In the words of one tester, 'the girl is now like a rotten potato', who must be kept away from virgin girls in order not to 'spoil the bunch'.[104]

Women as 'mothers of this world'

Women's roles as mothers and caregivers are central to understanding womanhood. As one mother said, 'Women are responsible, because the woman, they don't want to see other people dying of AIDS, because we are mothers of this world.'[105]

It is regularly reported that women take responsibility for caring for the sick and dying in the home – a task made more difficult when they themselves are HIV-infected. In addition, 'There is evidence to suggest that women's physical and psychological security might be compromised due to a lack of support within the household.'[106] A lot of AIDS health-care programmes rely on home-based care. In Alexandra, north of Johannesburg, the lack of involvement of men has limited the holistic provision of HIV care and support. 'Men were simply not interested in providing what was seen to be a woman's role for caring and support of sick people. Even those men who were active restricted their activities to more practical tasks such as managing the other volunteers and distributing food parcels.'[107]

Similar findings were reported in KwaZulu-Natal. The devastating impact of HIV on women's health in this community has made it almost impossible for them to act as caregivers and their male partners are often not willing to look after them.

My client came to visit me at the Friends-for-Life offices. She then informed me of her sad news, that her boyfriend has chased her away. She said when she arrived at home her boyfriend was with another woman at their place. He chased her away and refused to allow her to enter the house. When her sister heard the sad news, she rushed to find out what has really happened. The boyfriend explained that she is always sick and he can't take it anymore … he needs a woman who will take care of him.[108]

Women also face the terrible predicament of transmitting HIV to their babies either during childbirth or through breast-feeding. Because HIV testing takes place routinely at antenatal clinics, many women only learn of their HIV-positive status when they are pregnant. Thirty per cent of babies born to HIV-positive women are infected. This could be halved with a single dose of Nevirapine given to the mother during labour and to the baby shortly after birth. However, owing to government policy, this medicine has until recently not been made available to women, who can't afford to buy it themselves. The impact of the loss that many women have to bear is immense. 'I got a baby in August 1996. My child started to get sick in December '96. The child became sick badly and died in April '97. After the child died, my boyfriend fell sick in May 1997. He experienced complications and died.'[109]

The total lack of support for women coping with illness and death of family members due to HIV/AIDS seriously undermines their position within the household.

Women bear the brunt of the HIV/AIDS epidemic in South Africa. Not only are they more vulnerable to infection but they also carry the burden of care for their families. Understanding women's sexuality and unequal gender relations is thus an important part of making sense of HIV/AIDS in South Africa.

(Right) An AIDS patient is taken care of by her niece, who was taught by the South Coast Hospice how to care for her aunt

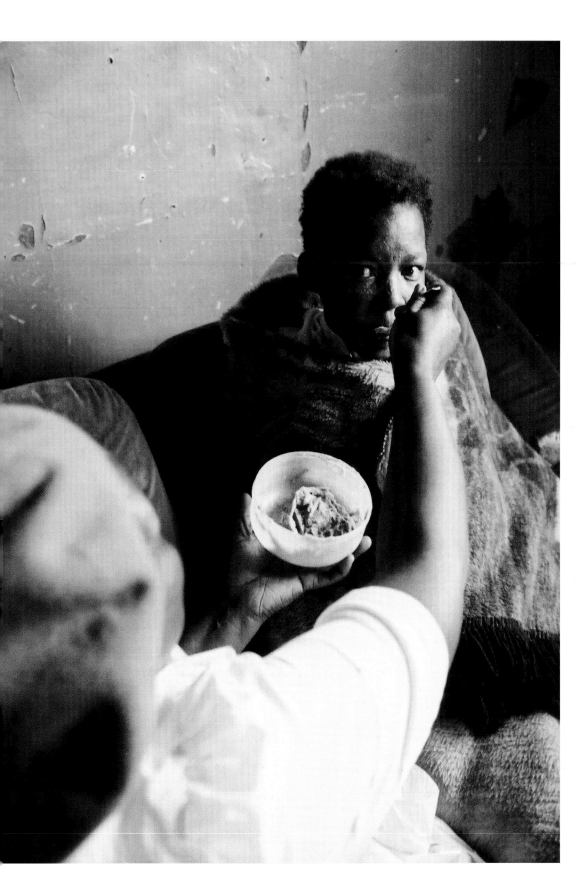

BEING A CHILD IN SOUTH AFRICA

Of course there's the fact that in Southern Africa, (mainly black) youth routinely and from young ages have to perform adult tasks and assume adult roles. The entire construct of youth becomes problematic.[110]

A very high proportion of the South African population is under the age of 20 years. This amounts to eighteen million people or 44% of the population. Young people are a vulnerable group in terms of access to education, employment, housing and health. They are also particularly vulnerable to HIV infec-tion (especially young girls). In 1998, according to the national antenatal sero-prevalence survey, 21% of women under the age of 20 tested HIV positive. This was double the 1997 figure of 12.7%, and was by far the largest increase in any age group.

Young people are also affected by other STIs. A substantial proportion of the four million cases reported each year occur amongst adolescents and young adults. STIs make young people more vulnerable to HIV infection. Research shows that people are becoming sexually active at an earlier age. This is borne out by teenage pregnancy sta-

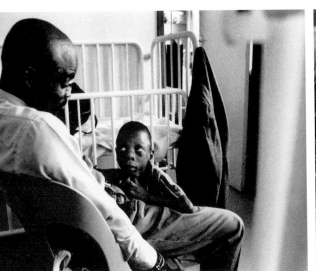

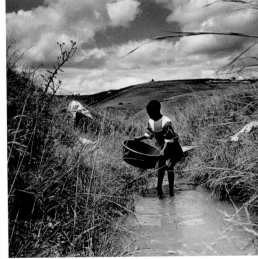

Aids takes its toll in infant mortality

Hundreds of tiny coffins bear witness to the extent of fatal disease

Bongiwe Nzimande this week buried her grandson, Sinemandla, who died eight days after he was born. 'It was a shortage of blood,' she said, after performing the final rites at his funeral. 'He just couldn't breathe.'

Sinemandla is among 372 babies who have been buried at the Azalea and Mountain Rise Cemeteries in Pietermaritzburg. Health officials and undertakers this week said that although AIDS is not a notifiable disease by law, they believed that most of the 372 babies could have died of AIDS-related illnesses.

When the *Sunday Times* visited the Azalea Cemetery this week, nine tiny coffins were being offloaded for paupers' burials. Pietermaritzburg's senior cemetery superintendent, Ziggy Maphanga, confirmed that 372 babies were buried at both cemeteries between April and August this year. 'Like the 990 infants that were

tistics. In 1995, 31% of girls reported that they had dropped out of school owing to unplanned pregnancy. In fact, teenage pregnancies accounted for one-third of all live births in South Africa in the same year.

The culture of crime and violence also affects young people, with a significant proportion of sexual abuse occurring among adolescents.[111] The media have recently highlighted the sexual abuse of school children and the growing incidence of child rape. According to police crime statistics, between January and December 2000, 13 540 children under 17 years were raped, 7 899 of whom were under the age of 11.

There is no doubt that the AIDS epidemic has significantly changed the nature of childhood. Historically, children living in poorer communities have always assumed adult responsibilities, such as domestic work, child care (of siblings), and contributing to the household income. In households where parents are sick and dying, the burden on children is immense, and South Africa is currently facing an unprecedented growth in the number of child-headed households.

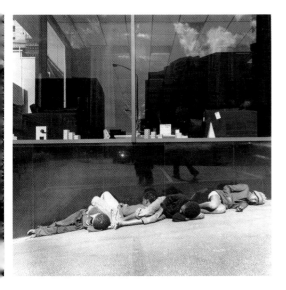

(From left to right)

A young HIV-positive boy holds onto his father's legs as they share a brief moment at the Cotlands Baby Sanctuary

A girl washing clothes in a stream outside Port Shepstone, KwaZulu-Natal

Street children in central Cape Town

buried here last year, most of the children this year died of HIV/AIDS,' he said. Robert Pawinski, from the KwaZulu-Natal Department of Community Health, said that the infant mortality rate had gone up a worrying degree. Pawinski said a recent study found that between 70% and 80% of children suffering from pneumonia were HIV positive.

Steven Naick, a senior manager at Pietermaritzburg's Parks and Recreation Division, said, 'In an area of over 150 graves, there are only two people who are over the age of 60.

The rest are people between the age of 20 and 30 years old.' Naick said there had been a dramatic increase in paupers' burials. 'Many people are requesting pauper burials for their dead. It's because of the stigma attached to families that have loved ones who have died of AIDS.'

Michael Zuma, a gravedigger at Azalea, said he digs about 40 graves during the week and between 35 to 50 over weekends for burials. 'But by Monday, they are full. Most of these graves are for babies who have died of AIDS.'[112]

Defining childhood and adolescence

According to psychologists, childhood spans the years from six to puberty. This is a critical stage for children to develop intellectually, socially and physically. It is a time when they should be encouraged to experience childhood fully and be allowed to encounter their environments free of adult responsibility. Adolescence (usually the teenage years) is a turbulent time, when young people develop a sense of their own identity as distinct from their parents. It is also a time of engaging with and making sense of the world around them. It is a time of social and sexual experimentation. These are broad categorisations but ones that provide a useful framework for thinking about childhood and adolescence. The experience of childhood is important for laying the foundation for the way men and women behave as adults. It is in childhood that ideas about gender relations and sexuality are formed.

The boundaries between different age groups are of course fluid and context-specific. In South Africa, the definition of childhood has always been unclear. For example, children and young people have been at the forefront of political struggle. Also, conditions of extreme poverty have resulted in children assuming adult responsibilities very early in life. HIV/AIDS has exacerbated this as an increasing number of children face life without their parents.

The changing context of sexual initiation

Rural children were particularly vulnerable to abuse as many were raped doing isolated

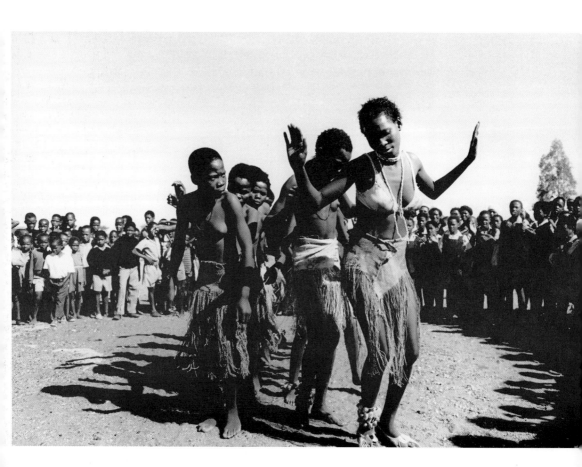

domestic chores, such as collecting wood or water. 'Parents also leave children unattended at home during the day, believing neighbours will look after them.'[113]

Sexual initiation is occurring at a much younger age than in the past and is often coercive. In a study of rural areas in the Eastern Cape, some 22% of young respondents had had sexual intercourse at or below the age of 11. The context within which young people have sex has changed dramatically over the past century. The nature of early sexual experimentation has changed radically.[114] In the past, the power of adolescent sexuality in rural areas was traditionally acknowledged and controlled by elders in the community. This was done through non-threatening forms of sex such as thigh sex or non-penetrative sex, which

More than five million children in South Africa – 30% of those under the age of seventeen – regularly go hungry, according to an IDASA study. A quarter of the country's very poor children are in KwaZulu-Natal, and a further quarter in the Eastern Cape. Mpumalanga and Limpopo are home to a share of 10% each. The study says that 59% (10.5 million) of the eighteen million children below the age of 17 are poor, in that they lack income. At most, only 12% of South Africa's poor children were receiving social security in the form of child-support grants (of R110 a month per child under the age of 6 and care dependency grants of R570 a month for children with severe disabilities).[115]

(Left) A puberty dance, Kuruman, Northern Cape

(Right) Morris Isaacson School, Soweto

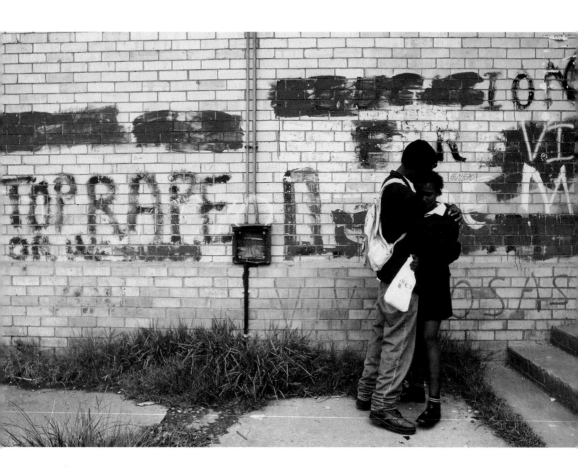

A third of children leaving school this year will have been the victims of some form of sexual abuse, according to an independent study conducted by CTI Africa. If the child attends a school in the Western Cape or Gauteng, the figure is likely to be higher. Dr Neil Andersson, an international epidemiologist who led the research, says, 'It is well into epidemic proportions. In a class of 40 children, two will admit to having been raped in the past year.' The report turned up surprisingly high incidences of sexual violence against males. One in 20 boys of school age admitted to being sexually abused either by an older male or female or by gangs of girls of school age. But it is not considered acceptable for boys to admit abuse so such cases are not being publicised. Children in focus groups said that the police would laugh if boys reported that they had been raped. The majority of people believed that women were to blame for being abused and 15% of girls and 20% of boys believed that it was unacceptable to refuse to have sex with a boyfriend. The study showed that schoolgirls would often have the same cavalier attitudes towards sex as men between the ages of 35 and 50, suggesting that adults are passing on dysfunctional beliefs.

'Child abuse is a hidden epidemic but my guess is people in communities know about it. It is not that hidden,' said Andersson. It occurs in all economic bands and more than half the abusers are known by the children. 'The problem', he says, 'is getting worse because abusers know that they can get away with it.'[122]

helped young people to avoid unwanted pregnancies and STIs. This is in strong contrast to present norms, where they are often left to negotiate sexual mores on their own.

Teenage pregnancy is a big risk. One in three girls in South Africa will be pregnant before the age of 20.[116] So young people tend to see protective measures in terms of pregnancy prevention rather than STIs. The role of injectable contraceptives is pertinent in this regard as this method of contraception offers no protection against STIs. It also places responsibility for birth control squarely on the shoulders of young girls.[117]

Forced sexual initiation at an early age is one of the most significant factors in subsequent sexual development and practice.[118] Coercive sex happens so frequently that it has come to be seen as normal and is even accepted as part of having sex by both girls and boys. In a situation where sex is not associated with intimacy it may also be seen as a resource to be transacted. Researchers point to the high levels of violence associated with sexual relationships amongst young people. Girls are often afraid to speak about this violence because they are not supposed to be having sex.

More young people are having sex now than in the past,[119] and there are often extreme age differences between the initiated and the initiator.[120] Older male relatives, family friends and men in positions of power and influence, such as teachers, often sexually abuse young women. 'Sugar daddies' may entice young girls into sexual relationships in exchange for necessities or 'treats'. These men are generally older and economically independent and therefore have considerable power and access to girls.[121] The girls face an increased risk of HIV exposure because of the unequal power relations between them and their partners and the fact that older men generally have larger sexual networks. The threat of violence makes condom negotiation extremely difficult. Also, the expectation that children should be able to negotiate sex safely is inappropriate and impossible.

An extreme environment where young people are particularly vulnerable to violent and coercive sex is that of closed institutions. A number of young people pass through prisons and reformatories, in which there are high levels of sexual violence. AIDS-related deaths in prisons are estimated to have increased by 80%. There has been a 584% increase in prison deaths from 'natural causes' over the past five years (from 186 deaths in 1995 to 1087 in 2000).[123]

Attitudes to sex

Unequal gender relations have a big influence on attitudes to sex among young boys and girls. For instance, boys often expect sexual intercourse to be an integral part of relationships. One study on condom use amongst secondary school pupils found that 'males feel that the normal duration of a relationship before sex is seven days, whereas girls will stay in a relationship for more than a month before having sex'.[124] Not only is there an expectation that relationships will be sexual but coercion is seen as an acceptable part of sexual conduct.[125]

Peer groups are very important in developing attitudes towards sex. One study shows how gangs and politicised youth influence sexual socialisation.[126] Peer pressure amongst boys places a premium on power and control over girls – their movements, behaviour and sexual availability.

Boys have a sense of undisputed power over their girlfriends; that is, they feel they have control over them. They think that love is synonymous with sex. Like men, boys consider 'love' to mean access to sexual intercourse

with their girlfriends.[127] As one researcher says, 'common to both young men and women is the belief that a man has a right, or even a duty, to force himself onto a women who displays reluctance and shyness.'[128] Being HIV positive does not change these practices and a number of studies point to the fact that young people often don't perceive themselves to be at risk.

Shared beliefs are important amongst youth.[129] They are particularly important when they reinforce prevailing power relations between boys and girls. One of the most prevalent beliefs is that youth is a time of irresponsibility. In other words, it is not a time to discuss safer sex and HIV/AIDS. In this way, shared beliefs influence sexual activity and work against safer-sex practices. Trust in sexual relationships also influences young people's attitudes to sex and condom use. The use of condoms may suggest a lack of trust in a partner.

Using condoms gets in the way of 'youthful romance' and can be a source of embarrassment and discomfort. Condoms are seen as unnatural. The idea of 'natural sex' also accounts for young people's negative attitudes towards masturbation. When the subject of masturbation was raised in role-plays amongst youth in the Durban area, the discussions resulted in 'awkwardness, laughter, and stigma from those putting forward a view'.[130]

AIDS orphans and child-headed households

Two-thirds of the 16.3 million children in South Africa live below the poverty line. A fifth of children in South Africa do not live with their mothers. It is estimated that by 2015 almost 12% of South African children will be orphans as a result of HIV/AIDS. South Africa is seeing increasing numbers of children in distress – a situation made worse by the collapse of traditional models of child care such as the extended family. Rising unemployment levels mean that fewer and fewer adults are in a position to provide for the household. Adults in the prime of their working lives are also most vulnerable to HIV infection.[131] This places a substantial financial and emotional burden on grandparents, who have increasingly become the prime guardians of these children. A case study of a foster-care pilot project in Bushbuckridge in Limpopo Province suggested that there is a need to identify workable models to ensure that children are properly integrated into the community.[132]

In situations where the deceased person is a single parent, many orphans suffer a double loss because they are often unable to remain in the care of a family member. These orphans require emotional and psychological support that is not available in poor communities. Mental health services are unavailable, overcrowded or unaffordable. However, innovative ways of helping children to deal with trauma have been developed and piloted. One project documented the use of memory boxes as a way of building up resilience in orphans and traumatised children in KwaZulu-Natal.

Orphans have to manage the family resources and assume adult responsibilities at a very young age. The burden of responsibility for looking after siblings often rests with the eldest female child. The South African Department of Welfare has recognised the growing problem of child-headed households by changing the law to allow under-age youth to access child-support grants. However, in order to successfully claim these grants children need important documentation such as birth and death certificates and identity documents. In sub-Saharan Africa, where 70% of births are not registered, children often fall through the welfare safety net.

Being a child in South Africa does not match the realities of childhood in countries not experiencing the ravages of HIV/AIDS. Far from it. Children are increasingly vulnerable as parents die on an unprecedented scale. Children are more susceptible to HIV infection through violence and abuse. Measures to protect them are inadequate. Family structures are also being stretched to breaking because of the assumption that extended families will absorb the growing number of AIDS orphans.

Memory boxes serve as a way of remembering parents who have died of HIV/AIDS. The first step in compiling a memory box is for facilitators to do an oral history interview with surviving family members. This is transcribed in a way that is easy to read, especially for children. This interview forms the basis of the booklet. Often, even in extremely poor families, photographs are kept in the house; these are copied by those facilitating the process and later included in a booklet along with photographs of places which remind children of their parents. The final memory box includes: the box, decorated by the children; the booklet containing the story of the deceased parent(s); the tape-recording of the interview; photographs of parents or family members; any object evoking the memory of the parents.[133]

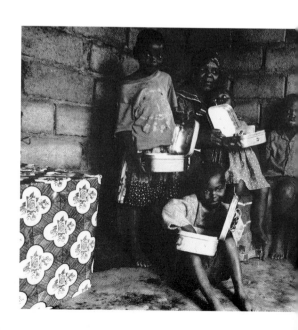

CONCLUSION

The HIV/AIDS epidemic in Southern Africa is mostly driven by the distinctive and dramatic interaction of sex, gender and power relations.

We have seen that masculinity is a critical area of inquiry when it comes to understanding the course of the AIDS pandemic in South Africa. The combined effects of common male behaviour, such as having multiple sexual partners, exercising control over women, engaging in coercive sex, violence between men, and the use of alcohol and drugs, are a large part of the problem.

However, the HIV/AIDS epidemic has led to a greater understanding of sexuality and gender relationships in South Africa. In trying to understand how the virus has been transmitted in the region, researchers have developed a better understanding of sex and the power relationships that exist between men and women. In some cases this new knowledge has challenged old orthodoxies and stereotypes. Research that reveals the pressures (particularly financial ones) that men experience in order to please women starts to unseat more common ideas about women as victims in relationships. So too does research that highlights the strategies women adopt to ensure their survival.

Childhood has also been re-examined in light of the fact that children are most vulnerable to HIV infection and to the social and economic consequences of the epidemic. Changes in family structure and the roles that children have to play in the absence of parental authority are new and urgent priorities for research.

The interconnection of sex and power with broader social and economic factors also extends our understanding of the HIV/AIDS epidemic. Making sense of sex and sexual practices is not just about understanding individual choices and values. More fundamentally, it is about understanding the society in which we live. In many respects the disease is invisible because of social stigma. But the research on HIV/AIDS has revealed a great deal about sex, sexuality and gender relations in Southern Africa.

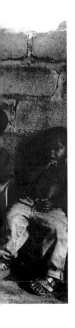

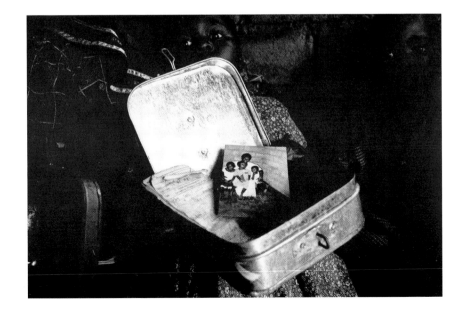

'AN EPIDEMIC WAITING TO HAPPEN'

Social disruption and social change

The health risks of mining and migrancy

Epidemics in historical perspective

Owning the epidemic – a history of moral panic and racial stereotyping

Reclaiming cultural traditions

AIDS – an apartheid illness?

The transition to democracy

Why has HIV/AIDS exploded in some regions of the world, while remaining dormant or contained in others?[134] How do we explain the exponential growth of the AIDS epidemic in South Africa that took place in the 1990s? The prevalence of HIV in South Africa was less than 1% in 1990 and by 2000 rose to 24%. In order to answer these questions we need to go back in time. Looking at the past will give us an insight into the way South African society has developed and the impact this has had on the HIV/AIDS epidemic.

Medical scientists provide biological explanations for the progression of the epidemic. They ask: is the virus different in Africa? What role do co-factors such as STIs play in the creation of explosive epidemics? For social scientists the explanation lies in social processes and structures. They ask questions like: how have social factors promoted HIV/AIDS? What is the role of the migrant labour system in the spread of HIV/AIDS? How have other epidemics shaped the AIDS crisis? What is the role of poverty in the transmission of the virus? Why are more women than men HIV positive? Why have people not changed their sexual behaviour in order to curb the epidemic? To what extent has the struggle against apartheid and the transition to democracy shaped the epidemic?

South Africa is a classic 'high risk situation' – a phrase coined to describe a context in which HIV/AIDS will thrive. At the beginning of the epidemic, the term 'high risk groups' was commonly applied to homosexuals, drug users and sex workers because it was thought that AIDS affected these groups in particular. As epidemiological understanding of the disease grew and everybody was seen to be at risk, the term 'high risk group' was replaced with 'high risk behaviour'. Both these terms stigmatise people and blame individuals. Neither takes into account the overriding importance of social context and how life circumstances and environment substantially shape one's risk of infection.

South Africa has a complex social history, fraught with conflict and characterised by sweeping change. AIDS is by no means the first epidemic to strike South Africa. During the course of the 20th century hundreds of thousands of South Africans died of smallpox, Spanish flu, TB and STIs. The virulence of these epidemics, combined with limited access to health care, had a devastating impact on the health of the population. AIDS is, however, unique in several ways. Biologically, the illness progresses very slowly, with few, if any, apparent symptoms. There is also no vaccine and no cure. Its unique combination of attributes makes AIDS unlike any plague human beings have had to contend with in the past.

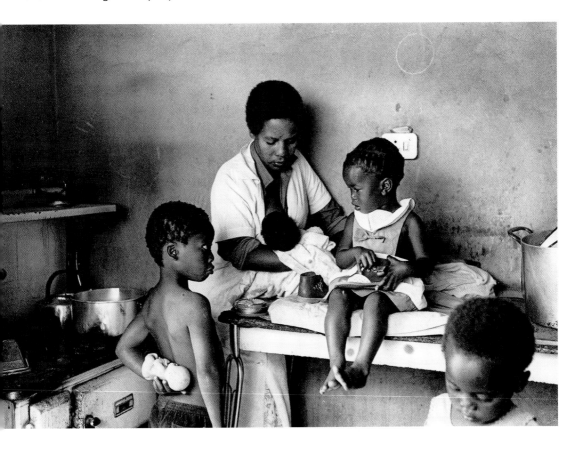

SOCIAL DISRUPTION AND SOCIAL CHANGE

What have industrialisation and urbanisation, population migration and the migrant labour system got to do with the AIDS epidemic in South Africa? How have prior epidemics and regional conflicts affected AIDS? These aspects of history are very relevant to the AIDS epidemic in South Africa. Reflecting on the syphilis epidemic in South Africa during the 1930s and '40s, Dr Sidney Kark said:

Without an understanding of the economic factors involved and the historical factors of the vast social pathological changes brought about during the last seventy years, no treatment will save the spread of syphilis in South Africa. Treatment of individuals … cannot succeed in any but a few cases. The first line of treatment must be to remedy the unhealthy social relationships which have emerged as the inevitable result of masses of men leaving their homes every year …[135]

Kark alerted us to the central importance of social disruptions in the spread of disease, in particular the movement of young men to the cities and away from their families of origin in rural areas.

The discovery of gold and diamonds in the late 19th century created an intense and growing demand for labour. Pre-existing forms of migrancy, where young men travelled far from their homes to work on white farms, were transformed into a vast system of labour mobilisation. Initially this system was shaped by continuing political and economic independence. But over time, conquest, the loss of land, taxation and recruiting monopolies left migrants and their communities with little room to manoeuvre. Migrant labour became the basis of a cheap labour system that left deep scars on the region.

Part of the appeal of migrant labour to both employers and the state was that workers' families remained in rural areas. While men

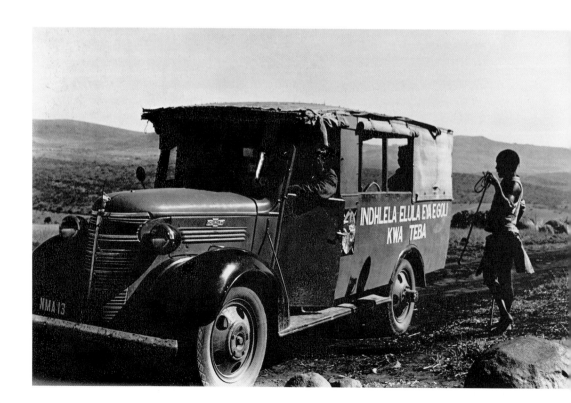

sent home some of their wages, their families also depended heavily on local resources for housing and subsistence. Many migrants who viewed urban areas as uncivilised, disease-ridden and dangerous places also saw migrancy 'as a necessary evil which had to be undertaken not only in order to pay taxes but also to secure the resources to marry, build a homestead, accumulate cattle and ultimately to allow for rural retirement'.[136]

In many countries around the world migrant labour occurred mainly during periods of economic transition, prior to workers and their families settling permanently in the cities. But in South Africa it has been the main source of labour to the mines for over a hundred years and has played a critical role in the wider development of industry. Migrant workers were drawn, not only from the rural areas of South Africa, but from a range of other countries in the region. They worked in mines, factories and offices, on farms, and as domestic workers. Critical con-

(Left) Recruiting for mine labour in the rural districts of South Africa in the early 20th century

(Right) Migrant workers arriving in Johannesburg in the 1950s

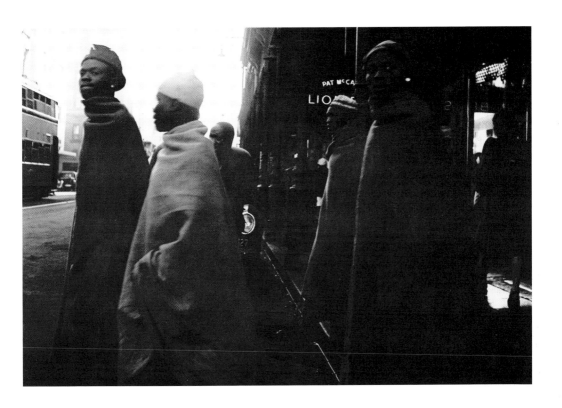

sequences of this system included a constant flow of people between rural and urban areas, and large concentrations of single men living far from their families for long periods of time.

The long-term separation of migrant men from their wives and families, along with the ever-present dangers of mining work and other high-risk, low-paid jobs (such as in foundries), helped foster aggressive masculinities and sexualities among migrant labourers. These in turn have contributed massively to the rapid spread of HIV/AIDS.

As a study of Basotho migrants on the gold mines of Carletonville in the 1990s observes, 'masculinity emerged as a master narrative penetrating informants' accounts of their more specifically health-related behaviour.' The study characterised masculinity as comprising two principal sets of features. On the one hand were notions of 'bravery, fearlessness and persistence in the face of the demands of underground work' (and, one might add, other men's violence on the mines). On the other hand was masculine sexuality, which one of the study's informants expressed in a particularly striking sentiment when he observed, 'There are two things to being a man: going underground and going after women.'

Linked to such masculine sexualities were 'repertoires of insatiable sexuality, the need for multiple partners and a manly desire for the pleasure of flesh-to-flesh sexual contact', all of which 'made migrant mine workers especially vulnerable to HIV infection'.[137] The study perceived such masculinities as culturally constructed – a mechanism to cope with life on the mines.

The explosive spread of STIs, especially syphilis, in the urban and rural areas of black South Africa earlier in the 20th century, is often attributed to similar attitudes among migrant labourers at the time. More recently, individuals infected with STIs have been much more susceptible to contracting

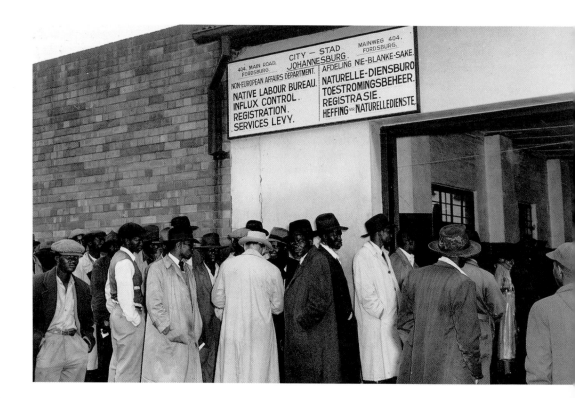

HIV/AIDS, and this has greatly aggravated the epidemic. Migrant labour undoubtedly contributes massively to the spread of HIV/AIDS in the 21st century. However, the connection between syphilis and migrant labour was not always present. This alerts us to the critical importance of social and cultural factors in promoting or inhibiting the spread of STIs. It must be emphasised that cultural and social factors cannot be totally divorced from material circumstances. Nevertheless they can attain a certain latitude and a capacity for improvisation which is partly independent from the exigencies of daily survival. Such cultural and behavioural creativity is thus one hope for containing HIV/AIDS.

The study of Basotho migrants highlights the impact of 'macho' masculinities and aggressive male sexualities among late-20th-century migrant miners on sexual relations and the spread of STIs and HIV/AIDS. This close association has not always existed, certainly not in the towns. The accentuation

(Left) Reporting to the Labour Bureau in Johannesburg, mid-20th century

(Right) Men sharing a room in a mine hostel, Rustenburg, late 20th century

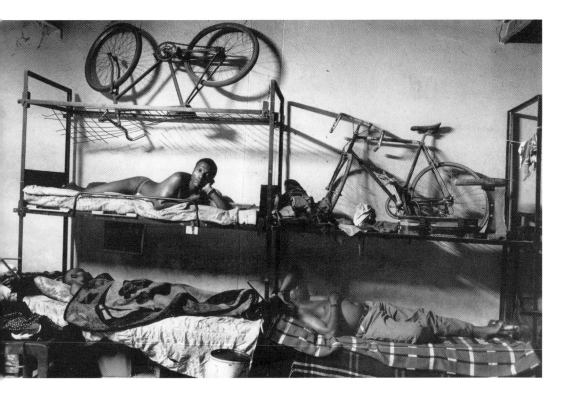

of aggressive risk-taking masculinities seems to be intimately bound up with the experience of migrant labourers on the mines. Another researcher recounts the allure of the regime of violence in early 20th-century mines, what is appositely termed this 'world without women'.[138] Others have described Basotho shaft sinkers' self-celebration of their brave, risk-taking physically powerful masculinities in the 1930s, 1940s and probably earlier.[139] Some researchers explicitly connect new forms of violent masculinities among the youth culture of the *indlabini* in parts of the Transkei to the experience of migrant labour.[140]

Yet aggressive masculinity and predatory aggressive sexuality have not always gone together. As labour migrancy was elaborated into a tightly regimented migrant-labour system in South Africa at the beginning of the 20th century, societies exporting migrant workers responded creatively to their new circumstances by fashioning new migrant cultures. The core values of these cultures were instilled in boyhood. Teenage boys on the cusp of adulthood were required to spend extended periods of time in initiation or circumcision lodges. The lessons learned in these lodges were rarely forgotten. Among the central moral and social injunctions hammered home in these periods of socialisation was an absolute prohibition on liaisons with urban women. Apart from death, the loss of young men to the siren calls of African women in the towns was the primary threat to rural societies caught up in the migrant labour system. Thus the ban on associating with urban women was a core component of every migrant culture. Examples abound, and we cite only one. Here the speaker is Lebike Mothubatse:

Our elders did not permit that you, a child having come to the town, should desire [urban women. They said] you will die soon. The women of the towns kill people. It was a binding regulation [and if you breached it] they would drive you out of the compound ... It was a disgrace ... they will just part ways with you.[141]

Migrant workers recognised that death was a possible consequence of sexual relations with urban women. They perceived these women as being riddled with STIs, including syphilis, which killed in its tertiary stages.

One way of channelling sexual desires was through non-penetrative homosexual relationships. This was especially common among migrants serving longer contracts on the mines, and has been extensively documented.[142] Later work on male–male marriages on the mines suggests that these relationships also reflected men's desire for close emotional ties and homely comforts, particularly among older, more senior men, who would take on new male recruits as wives to minister to their needs.[143] The general effect of these cultural practices was to curb the spread of STIs.

Despite these rigid moral prescriptions (largely unknown to early medical practitioners) STIs, particularly syphilis, were perceived to be rampant in the early 20th century in the Cape and in large parts of the Transvaal. The Contagious Diseases Commission of 1906 claimed that 75–80% of the people in these areas 'were syphilitics'. The diamond and gold mines and migrant labour were generally blamed for the spread of STIs. The railway was seen as the harbinger of the epidemic, facilitating its national spread. Naturally unrestrained and promiscuous sexual behaviour among African migrants and the pool of African prostitutes that had gathered in the industrial areas were held to be the cause.

By the early 1930s, however, the medical establishment was beginning to realise that a large number of infections previously identified as venereal or congenital syphilis were in fact a related pre-existing African disease, which was not sexually transmitted, and was given the name of endemic syphilis. Few, however, admitted or recognised the corollary of this finding – that migrant cultures generally exercised strong sexual discipline and that migrancy was not solely responsible for the spread of STIs.[144]

Nevertheless, venereal syphilis did spread until it reached near-epidemic proportions after the Second World War. How did this happen? By the 1920s the Public Health Department estimated that about 10% of the African population had venereal syphilis. As late as 1930 a survey of mine recruits found low rates of venereal syphilis in the primary labour recruiting areas in South Africa (Transkei and Ciskei) and median rates in the middle-range labour-exporting area of Basutoland. From then on, rates of venereal syphilis climbed in Transkei, Ciskei, the Eastern Transvaal, Basutoland and Natal. Generally the route of infection was via migrants returning from the towns. Something had changed.

The most important development during the 1930s and 1940s was the rise of urbanisation. This was partly due to the growth of secondary industries and the tertiary service sector in the towns, which in some cases preferred more stable urban-rooted labour. Even then the great majority of 'urban' workers retained roots and families in the countryside. Many of them lived in single male quarters and remained, in some senses, migrant.[145]

An additional and critical component of urbanisation was the movement of rural women to the towns. This gathered pace in the 1930s and 1940s: in these decades tens of thousands of women migrated to the main urban areas of South Africa. Two geographical areas were particularly pronounced in this process, Basutoland and the Ciskei. The main reasons for the exodus of women from these areas were the departure of migrant husbands or male relatives to urban areas for extended periods, lack of material support, shortages and lack of access to land (above all for widows and unmarried or abandoned women). By the mid-1940s over half of the women in the Ciskei supported themselves independently of their husbands. Dozens of young girls were widowed as a result of the huge age gap between them and their spouses. Others were abandoned by absconding migrant husbands or had borne children outside of marriage. All too frequently in such cases, they were thrown out of family homesteads by patriarchs unwilling to support them and their offspring.

Single women grasped at straws. Some had children who sent home money and (much later) the old lived on pensions. Younger women faced a bleak future. As fertility lost its value, sexuality gained in importance. Many women came under pressure to take a lover in return for favours such as representation before a village council or the ploughing of her field.[146]

Promiscuity of this sort fostered the spread of STIs. Venereal diseases in maternity cases at Mount Coke Hospital grew from 1% of patients in 1938 to over 20% in 1948.[147]

Prior to the apartheid government's imposition of tighter influx control in the early to mid-1950s, many rural women preferred to flee to the towns. In 1940 one-sixth of adult women were absent from their homes in the Ciskei and living in the towns.[148] In Basutoland the figures were even more striking. By the late 1930s more than a quarter of the female population was absent from the territory.[149]

But few waged jobs were available for women in the towns. On the Witwatersrand and in Durban, for example, young men dominated even domestic work until the 1940s. Women arriving in the towns often entered into transient relations with men and survived by brewing illicit liquor. Many engaged in a variety of sexual transactions. Many of their clients were migrant men, who had either left or were considering leaving the enclosed world of the mines for higher-paying jobs and alternative accommodation in the towns. In these circumstances there was an explosion of venereal infections that were carried by migrants to their rural homes. When squatter camps, both unregulated and municipally regulated, began to grow and multiply in the 1940s a whole variety of sexually and non-sexually transmitted diseases spread unchecked.

The rapid spread of STIs can thus be identified with the intersection of migrant labour and urbanisation. As rural women left for the towns migrant cultures began to fray at the edges. The sexualities of migrants on the margins of migrant culture and moving towards the urban world underwent a radical change. New migrants or ex-migrants

competed for the sexual favours of newly urbanised women.[150] It was at this point that macho migrant masculinities and newly aggressive migrant or ex-migrant sexualities fused. Here lies one root of the current AIDS epidemic.

To this day, migrant labour remains a distinctive feature of South African economic and social life. The number of mineworkers employed on gold mines peaked at 500 000 in 1985. Recent years have seen massive retrenchments; nevertheless, mines still employ approximately 350 000 men. Through a series of government reforms during the 1970s and 1980s conditions in the compounds improved considerably, but they are still overcrowded, dirty and unhealthy. In a recent study of Carletonville, the biggest gold-mining complex in the world, it was found that most mineworkers live in the ten single-sex hostels close to the mineshaft. Living conditions are basic, with between four and fifteen workers sharing a room. Each man lives in cramped conditions with no more than a bed and a locker to call his own.[151]

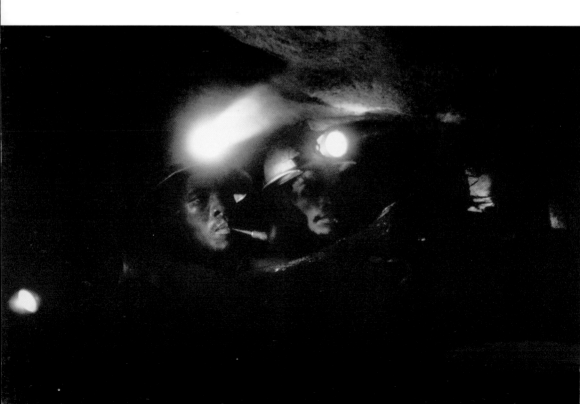

Not only are living conditions bleak, the mines are also extremely dangerous. In 1993, the Chamber of Mines documented that a mineworker has a 3% chance of being killed in a work-related accident and a 43% chance of suffering a reportable injury.

We have focused on migrancy and the mining industry because historically the majority of migrant workers have been employed in this sector. But other forms of migration are common across South Africa. Within a twelve-kilometre radius of Durban, for example, there are at least seven men's hostels with an excess of 43 000 officially registered beds, one women's hostel with over 1000 beds and one mixed hostel with 11 000 beds.[152] Similarly, from 1956 to 1966 the migrant population in Vosloorus, a township on the East Rand, grew from 12 261 to 25 386, accounting for 83% of the township population. By the early 1980s the township's municipal hostels alone accommodated nearly 18 000 men. The migrants were primarily employed in the industrial and manufacturing sectors.[153] Their living conditions were squalid and without privacy. As one migrant worker, Frans Photswane, described it:

It was an open hall and 16 of us lived in there. There was no dividing wall between the beds. We were just crammed in there like animals. The only furnishings … were a little locker, and small bed base without a mattress. As a rural boy I always felt ashamed of looking at naked elders … At times we were forced to go to other blocks to avoid looking at our own fathers, uncles and elder brothers undressed.[154]

Male circular migration is the predominant form of movement in South Africa but, as we have demonstrated, migration of young women is also common. For example, in a survey carried out in KwaZulu-Natal in 1996 it was found that 60% of men and about one-third of women between the ages of 19 and 49 were migrants.

At the peak of [the migrant labour system] in 1985, 1 833 636 South Africans were classed as migrants … that is, they were not regarded as resident in the areas where they worked. Of these, 771 397 came from the 'independent homelands' of Transkei, Bophuthatswana, Venda and Ciskei; and 1 062 239 from the 'self-governimg homelands' of Lebowa, Gazankulu, QwaQwa, KwaZulu, KwaNdebele and KaNgwane. However, South Africa's economic influence extended far beyond the country's borders. It was (and is) the richest country in the region, which meant that it drew in labour from as far away as Malawi and Angola. And this labour was needed. Despite the apartheid system there was not enough indigenous labour. In 1985, 27 814 Batswana, 139 827 Basotho, 30 144 Malawians, 68 665 Mozambicans and 22 255 Swazi were employed officially as migrants in South Africa. In addition there were many illegal migrants, mainly employed in the agricultural sector.[155]

THE HEALTH RISKS OF MINING AND MIGRANCY

Accidents and occupational injuries are obvious health risks associated with mining but they are not the only ones. In the early decades of the mining industry, workers died from pneumonia and meningitis, gastroenteritis, scurvy and lung diseases, including TB. Poor nutrition, crowded, damp conditions and sudden changes in temperature sapped the vitality of the miners, making them more susceptible to illness.

Migrancy drew large numbers of economically productive young men away from the rural economy and this had a negative impact on the health and well-being of the rural population.

South Africa's industrialisation was made possible by the constant movement of large numbers of sexually active men from town to countryside and back, bearing their diseases with them, resulting in the impoverishment of the countryside and the marginalisation of women and children ... For the vast majority it has spelt poverty and powerlessness.[156]

Overcrowding also undermined the health of those living in the African reserves. The 1913 and 1936 Land Acts entrenched the loss of land that African communities had experienced in the 19th century and demarcated a mere 13% of the total land mass of South Africa as reserves for Africans. As the population grew, these areas became severely overcrowded and resources such as water and land for grazing were depleted. In this context of reduced rural viability, nutritional failure and epidemic diseases had a dramatic impact on individuals, families and communities.[157]

Rural women were not simply the victims of male sexual promiscuity. In the absence of their partners they had sexual relations with other men or travelled to urban centres in search of money. A study of migrant men and their partners in northern KwaZulu-Natal shows that infection rates were higher amongst women than amongst returning migrants. The study questioned the circular migration thesis of urban–rural–urban HIV transmission and described a new pattern of HIV discordance (where only one partner is HIV positive). Preliminary data showed that in nearly 40% of discordant migrant couples the woman was infected and not the man. This finding highlights the importance of understanding the rural dynamics of the epidemic, and implies that successful prevention efforts should concentrate not only on the urban 'receiving areas' but on the rural 'sending areas' as well. It is important to study both ends of the migration spectrum at the same time.[158]

These findings support previous research showing that 2.3% of non-migrant rural women between the ages of 15 and 44 in KwaZulu-Natal were HIV positive, compared to 0.5% of men in the same age cohort.[159] Similarly, a study on the management of HIV/AIDS found that in HIV-discordant migrant couples it was often the woman who tested HIV positive.[160]

Transactional sexual exchanges can also play a decisive role in rural household economies, especially in cases where migrant-worker husbands have abandoned their wives.

Absent husbands who got involved in relationships in the city often did not send remittances back to the rural areas. During the nineteenth century, an abandoned woman could expect to be taken in by her kin but as the kinship systems began to break down, she had to go elsewhere. With the high rate of unemployment and the way in which gender relations were constructed, one of the few options available to these women was to become involved in relationships of sex in exchange for money and very often food and care. The most likely partner would be an unattached returning migrant – given that he would have some money to support her … the pattern of abandoned women was exacerbated by changes in marriage patterns as kinship structures began to crumble.[161]

Not all rural women could rely on regular remittances from the city. An important source of revenue for these women was the sale of beer, and their main customers were often returning migrants with ready cash. In this way some redistribution of money took place in the villages.[162] The sale of beer also offered opportunities for sexual liaisons.

The migrant-labour system created classic conditions for the spread of disease. It relied on the mass migration of virile, sexually active young men and formed new geographical and sexual networks (sexual highways) across the region. The disruption of family and social life brought about by industrialisation and migrancy created fertile conditions for the rapid spread of STIs. It is hardly surprising then that migrant mineworkers were amongst the first heterosexual men in South Africa to test positive for HIV infection in large numbers in the 1980s. This rang a particularly sombre alarm bell because of the danger of the epidemic spreading to large sections of the general population. For the first time it became clear that AIDS would be a heterosexual epidemic.

Shebeen in a rural district of the North West Province

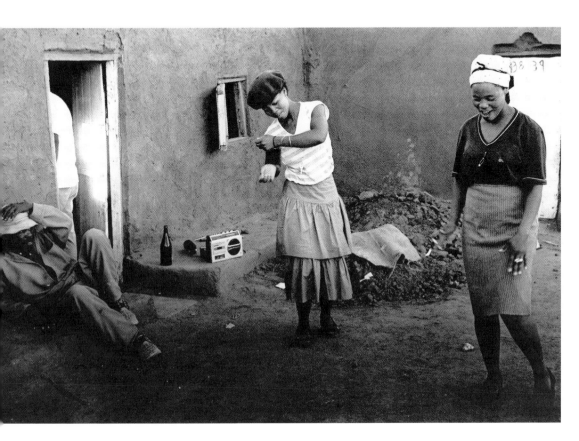

EPIDEMICS IN HISTORICAL PERSPECTIVE

What does history teach us about epidemics? Why is this information useful? There are strong historical similarities between the HIV/AIDS epidemic and others that have gone before it in South Africa. Yet there are also significant differences. It has been said that South Africa has never experienced an epidemic like HIV/AIDS. This is only partially true. AIDS is undoubtedly unique in several ways. The extraordinary speed with which the virus has travelled, its long period of dormancy, and the fact that it is a global disease affecting every part of the world make HIV/AIDS a distinctively modern epidemic. In biological terms too, AIDS is exceptional.

HIV has gone one better [than syphilis], by attacking and destroying the immune system which is itself supposed to fend off disease. People who have the virus have few if any obvious signs of infection, and may well be unaware of their infection, but can still pass it on to others, while the virus itself constantly changes, thus evading the armoury of the most sophisticated of modern drugs. All this makes it the ideal prefabricated killer.[163]

Howard Phillips, a medical historian, says:

HIV/AIDS is novel among South Africa's epidemics … its marrying of continuities from past epidemics with wholly new features is what is really distinctive about it. It does not stand outside of South Africa's epidemic past; it has grown out of it.[164]

What are the continuities from past epidemics? Smallpox, syphilis, Spanish flu and TB are just some of the major epidemics that happened in South Africa during the 19th and 20th centuries. However, little research has been done on the social history of epidemics in this country despite the dramatic impact they have had on the demographic make-up of our society, and the significant dents they have made in economic development. There is thus a tendency to exaggerate the unique and unprecedented character of AIDS because of the lack of historical perspective on epidemics generally.

TB has been described as the quintessential disease of poverty. Factors influencing its onset include malnutrition, physical stress, insufficient ventilation, overcrowding, and unsanitary conditions. In Britain TB declined

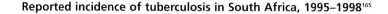

Reported incidence of tuberculosis in South Africa, 1995–1998[165]

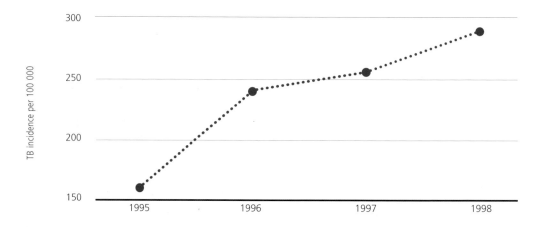

significantly before the introduction of the TB vaccination and antibiotics (in the 1950s), owing to a considerable improvement in public hygiene and social conditions.[166]

In 1933–34, the South African Department of Public Health launched a national campaign against TB, which recognised the role of poverty and other social ills in the spread of the disease.[167] For decades TB ravaged the poorer, more vulnerable sections of South African society. It was the most frequently occurring notifiable disease. In 1988, 98 000 cases of TB were reported. In 1997 the Medical Research Council estimated that South Africa had approximately 180 507 cases (55% reported). In other words, 419 of every 100 000 people had TB. Unlike HIV/AIDS, however, TB is preventable through vaccination and curable through medication.

TB has been directly implicated in the AIDS epidemic in a number of ways. People with HIV are susceptible to opportunistic infections, including TB, because their immune systems are depleted and they are less able to fight off infections. TB is a special case, though. One-third of South Africans are exposed to it as children. The primary infection remains dormant, and latent TB is reactivated by suppressed immunity associated with HIV. The TB epidemic has substantially increased the number of AIDS-related deaths because TB has a particularly debilitating effect on people with HIV. For example, the Medical Research Council shows that in 1997 33% of people with TB were probably also infected with HIV.[168] Parallels between AIDS and TB have also been drawn because vulnerability to HIV infection has been linked to poverty. In fact the epidemiology of TB is similar to that of AIDS.

But how is poverty implicated in the spread of HIV/AIDS? Poor people are more vulnerable to disease and ill health. In the period between the First and Second World Wars there was a general decline in African health. Malnutrition was widespread and morbidity rates for diseases associated with poverty were alarming. This was not just because of the lack of African health and medical services in urban and rural areas but also because of the socio-economic changes that were happening in South Africa.

Health and health care during the apartheid era left a legacy of inequitable and inadequate facilities. Preventable diseases were allowed to spread owing to low rates of vaccination, essential drugs were not widely available in the public health-care system and very few people had access to adequate curative care. Treatment of some diseases was given priority. During the early years of apartheid, if an epidemic broke out in 'non-white' areas and there was a fear that it would spread to white areas, strong measures were taken to prevent and eradicate the epidemic. STIs in particular were seen as a major threat and were managed with increased official zeal.

There are huge inequalities between the private and public health-care sectors. The majority of specialised health-care professionals such as general practitioners, dentists and pharmacists continue to work in the private health sector. The ratio of population to doctor is still four times greater in the public health sector than in the private health sector. And health-care facilities in the public sector, particularly in the rural areas, are wholly inadequate. This confirms that the inverse care law operates in South Africa, meaning that health services are most available to the people who need them least. Those who need health care the most have inadequate access to it.

Apartheid government policies have weakened community resilience. In the face of HIV/AIDS, communities often lack the social resources to manage and curb the spread of disease. This is referred to as 'social capital', which is defined as 'the existence of community networks, civic engagement (participation in these community networks), local identity and a sense of solidarity and equality with other community members, and finally, norms of trust and reciprocal help and support'.[169]

It has been widely argued that the presence of social capital is linked to positive health outcomes.[170] For example, the promotion of condom use and other safer-sex practices is most likely to succeed where young people feel that they are in command of their lives and are supported by trusted networks and positive role models. In a context where violence, substance abuse and social divisions are the order of the day, social cohesion and a sense of community are stifled and prevention programmes are unlikely to gain wide acceptance.

Poverty and its associated consequences, social disempowerment, and lack of access to health-care facilities and treatment for HIV infection hasten the spread of HIV in the most vulnerable sectors of society. But AIDS knows no boundaries. Wealth does not prevent infection, although having access to anti-retroviral drugs through the private health-care systems may stave off the onset of illness. The wealthier sector of society also has the ability to 'buy' a healthy lifestyle, including adequate nutrition, a good living environment and psychosocial networks of support.

It was the combination of these social factors and an environment of poor health that created the conditions in which, half a century later, the Human Immuno-Deficiency Virus was to flourish.

OWNING THE EPIDEMIC – A HISTORY OF MORAL PANIC AND RACIAL STEREOTYPING

In the 1930s and 1940s the public response to outbreaks of syphilis was one of panic. This panic had a strong racial theme.

Public fear over syphilis in the inter-war period may have grown out of, and to some extent displaced, earlier panics around rape scares and the 'black peril' that had gripped white society, particularly in the early years of the century. Both kinds of panic were the product of exaggerated fears. Both were driven by concern to protect the integrity of white bodies and by fears of African sexuality. The uproar over syphilis also reflected alarm at the growth of the black urban population and the proliferation of multi-racial slums. Behind these concerns lay anxieties about miscegenation and the fear of racial decline.[171]

Syphilis thus served to reinforce popular stereotypes amongst whites about black promiscuity and 'libidinous Africans'.[172] A parallel response and similar sets of stereotypes are attached to the transmission of HIV/AIDS. One of these stereotypes is that of the sexually promiscuous African male. It is this stereotype that so heavily informs the speech made by the South African president, Thabo Mbeki, late in 2001.

Thus does it happen that others who consider themselves to be our leaders take to the streets carrying their placards, to demand that because we are germ carriers, and human beings of a lower order that cannot subject its [sic] passions to reason, we must perforce adopt strange opinions, to save a depraved and diseased people from perishing from self-inflicted disease … Convinced that we are but natural-born, promiscuous carriers of germs, unique in the world, they proclaim that our continent is doomed to an inevitable mortal end because of our unconquerable devotion to the sin of lust.[173]

Mbeki's speech is an extreme response but it clearly echoes widely held white stereotypes about the relationship between African sexuality and STIs in apartheid and pre-apartheid South Africa. Responding to this historical legacy, Mbeki's re-manipulation of moral panic has served to close discussion on the racial and sexual patterns of HIV transmission. Ironically, the speech moralises about sexual behaviour in a climate where public health campaigns are encouraging open and frank discussion of sexual practices and mores.

Suspicions and stereotypes about the origin of the disease are equally widespread among Africans. For example, in 1991, the popular magazine *Drum* carried, without comment, an article entitled 'Is AIDS a Conspiracy against Blacks?', which reinforced the urban legend that AIDS was deliberately introduced to the African population in the dying days of apartheid. The decision of the director of the Highveld Blood Transfusion Service in 1990 not to accept blood from blacks or coloureds is a vivid example of how these stereotypes informed medical policy and practice.

There are many parallels between HIV/AIDS and other epidemics that occurred in South Africa during the 20th century. One of these is in the way governments have responded. Those infected and those seen to be responsible for the spread of disease have been blamed, punished and isolated. In the 1880s, for example, members of the Muslim community were forcibly quarantined for smallpox and members of the Natal Indian community for cholera. In 1899, the Transvaal government restricted the movement of Indians because they were seen as vectors of bubonic plague.

During the bubonic plague epidemic in 1901–03, the Cape government tried to forcibly move all Africans from central Cape Town and Port Elizabeth to the outskirts of these cities. In 1918, attempts were made to prevent Africans with symptoms of Spanish flu from travelling by train. During the typhoid epidemics of 1917–24 and 1933–35, all third-class African passengers travelling on trains from the Transkei were subject to compulsory deverminisation.[174] And during the 1940s and 1950s, 'diseased natives' were deported to rural areas, forced to have treatment or charged for 'failing to seek medical attention for syphilis'.[175]

Blaming has the effect of stigmatising illness and disease. It also creates categories of 'those who are at risk' and 'those who are not'. Those individuals or groups who fall into the 'not at risk' category assume wrongly that a disease or epidemic has nothing to do with them. This makes them vulnerable to infection because they do not take precautions against it. In the early 1980s the spread of HIV/AIDS was blamed on homosexual men, intravenous drug users and prostitutes. In this climate of blaming, stigmatising and finger-pointing no one took responsibility – no one owned the epidemic.

RECLAIMING CULTURAL TRADITIONS

Sexual norms, expectations and practices are the cornerstone of cultural values and beliefs. Where different expressions of culture clash, discussions about sexuality evoke passionate responses. Nowhere is this more evident than in the responses to the HIV/AIDS epidemic. The refrain 'It is not in our culture' is often used to justify behaviour that is sometimes contrary to public health messages and flies in the face of biomedical knowledge. South Africa has a well-resourced AIDS education campaign and knowledge of how HIV is transmitted is comparatively high amongst the general population. Yet the use of condoms, for example, is often rejected. One of the reasons for this lies in an invocation of 'traditional culture'.

One way that the past is romantically invoked is through the iconic figure of the polygamous patriarch – a figure who is often used to justify multiple sexual partners. Another example is the importance of fluid exchange during sexual intercourse, which is central to some men's cultural

taboo against the use of condoms. The high premium placed on women's fertility is another culturally shaped factor that prevents safer-sex practices.

But the notion of culture as circumscribing specific practices in spite of their serious health consequences is a static one. It suggests that culture is timeless and ahistorical. It does not accept that culture is dynamic and forever changing in response to internal pressures and external circumstances. In some respects, this desire to retain and recreate past traditions is a symptom of disempowerment and the fragmentation and disintegration of traditional society.

Sometimes the narrow appeal of 'It's not in our culture' draws on largely fictitious re-imaginings of the past. An historical study of sexual socialisation amongst South African youth questioned the contemporary assertion that parents do not talk to their children about sex because discussing intimate matters is not part of 'African culture'. In the 19th century, African communities were relatively open about sexual matters

Loverboys

Mr Ngcobo, along with two other middle-class men whom I spoke with, went on to challenge the way that today's men invoke the 'tradition' of *isoka*. These men did so by presenting more complex histories of *isoka*. In the past, they say, a good *isoka* used to have many girlfriends, but would intend to pay *lobola* (bridewealth). He would also be more content with the practice of *ukusoma* (to engage in non-penetrative thigh sex). But at that time there were also *isoka lamanyala* (*amanyala* was translated to me as meaning 'shit') who 'let women down' and transmitted diseases. This is likely to be an ideal distinction drawn up according to today's moral judgements. Indeed, one of the three men recalled how, when employed at the nearby paper mill SAPPI, he himself had many girlfriends, constantly re-contracting syphilis. He was an *isoka*, he says,

although he is less clear about whether he was a good one or a bad one. But the narrative disrupts the claims of an organic link between a single 'good' and 'traditional' *isoka* and today's *isoka* who has low-commitment sexual relations. This re-working of the past can have some unlikely allies. Within Mandeni, I noted how young township schoolgirls had a certain nostalgia for the lost era of 'love' ('*alusekho uthando*', there is no longer love). Their understanding, and very memories, of 'love' – constructed in part not only through family, schools and friends but through modern soap operas, magazines and music – nevertheless overlap with the older men's nostalgia. Together, they construct narratives of 'tradition' that disrupt modern meanings around *isoka*. Cultural processes never start with a blank sheet, but always rework actually existing meanings.[176]

although the extent to which parents actually spoke to their children directly is questionable. Adolescent sexuality was recognised as being particularly powerful and potentially destructive socially. Measures were therefore taken to regulate and control it. For example, thigh sex was socially sanctioned, whereas there were social proscriptions and penalties for penetrative sex.[177]

Knowledge of sex was an integral part of many African children's early sexual socialisation. This included sexual play amongst peers and learning from adults. As Godfrey Pitje, who grew up in Sekhukhuneland in the 1920s and 1930s, described:

As Pedi children usually sleep in the same room as their parents there can be no doubt that they are early instructed in sexual matters. They cannot help seeing the sexual performance of their parents. (Many adults also discussed sexual matters in the presence of their children). Not only do they learn about sex from such indiscreet conversation, but they also listen to quarrels in which whole lists of sexual obscenities and technicalities are recited.[178]

Historically there was a strong social taboo against teenage pregnancy. Researchers working in the Eastern Cape found that

Periodic inspections by elderly women were performed to see to it that the girls did not indulge in early sexual activity. There were also immediate negative consequences for those who broke the rules, e.g. once a girl fell pregnant her peers were all inspected and all the parents became extra vigilant towards their daughters' comings and goings. It was not only the said girl who had to bear the shame, but also the boyfriend, in that elderly women would come together, sing and march to the responsible boy's home to demand a fine in the form of livestock from the boy's family, in a process called *isihewula*. All this was done with much fanfare, and the boy's family not only had to pay immediately but also had to live with the shame their son had brought upon them.[179]

The introduction of Christianity to the South African hinterland drastically altered patterns of sexuality in the rural areas. There was a loosening of pre-existing sexual sanctions and an increase in premarital sex.[180]

Sex between the thighs: *hlobonga*

A 'man begins intercourse just within the vagina, the girl having her legs crossed, and when he feels he is going to pass semen, he draws away and passes on the girl's thighs. ... *Hlobonga* was a universal custom but it was one that must go on in secret. Every girl's mother, father and brothers know of this custom and that she would probably act in accordance with it, but woe betide her if she was caught by her elder brothers' ... [But even attempts to ban the practice by the Zulu king Cetshwayo in the 1870s failed] 'because ... girls and boys slept out in the open by stealth'. To enforce celibacy, elders sent chaperons, usually their older children, to supervise encounters between boys and girls ... [But] some homestead elders preferred any sexual activity to occur within their own homestead to discourage more serious transgression: 'a lover was allowed to *hlobonga* at the girl's home, a hut being set apart for the couple's use. An unmarried woman who had intercourse risked immediate censure from her family and perhaps prolonged ostracism. A girl who lost her virginity before marriage' knew she would of course lose value when the amount of *lobola* was being fixed.[181]

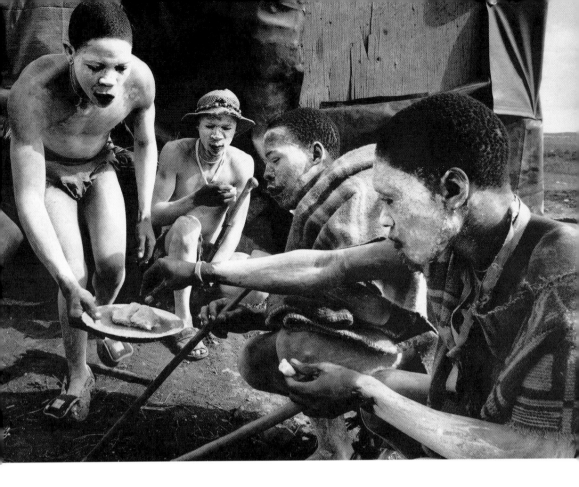

The disintegration of pre-Christian moral codes and sexual norms was also evident in Xhosa-speaking communities in the 1950s. 'Christian morality and the pursuit of modernity made a potent cocktail which stigmatised traditional forms of restraint but failed to curb the heightened sexual impulses of pubescent youths.'[182]

Distinctions were drawn between traditionalists (Red) and more modern Christians (School). 'Red' youth still went through initiation and were part of age groups whose sexual activity was monitored and regulated. However, such control and instruction did not exist within 'School' groups. In contrast to the open discussion of sex and sexual regulation within 'Red' communities, the subject was taboo in Christian communities, where youth were forbidden to engage in

premarital sex. 'Red people are open with their love affairs … the love affairs of a "Red" boy are even known to his mother. But I [a 'School' man] before I was twenty was even afraid to let my sisters know.'[183]

It appears that prior to the 1930s communities that had resisted the encroachment of Christianity were able to provide a better training for youth in matters of sexuality. But the degree of that success should not be overstated. These changes and disruptions in pre-Christian methods of sex education and youth socialisation were not limited to the rural areas. In the cities families experienced changes that influenced parental instruction and control. Increasing rates of teenage pregnancy and the formation of youth gangs became an unwelcome feature of some urban centres during the 1930s.

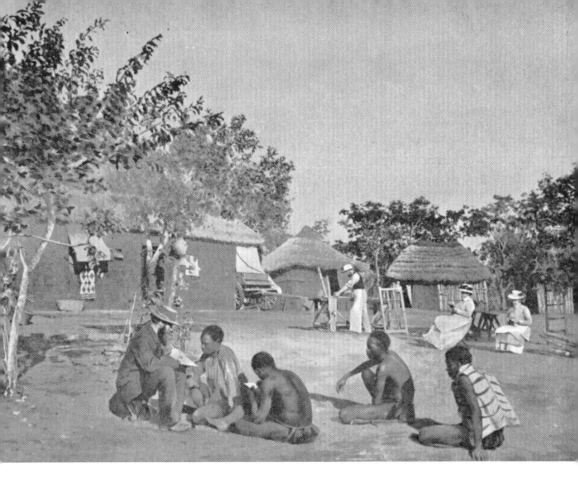

While black urban residents aspired to Western respectability, many – somewhat paradoxically – blamed the morally bankrupt city for the 'degeneration' of their youth and looked back nostalgically at indigenous African systems. This sort of contradictory attitude was epitomised in the popular Johannesburg newspaper, *Bantu World*. 'The temptations of youth [in the cities] are so much more varied than those of the rural areas,' it commented in a 1937 editorial article. Two years later it bemoaned the 'thousands of boys and girls growing up wild in the midst of the dazzling splendour of Western Civilisation, with its ... drinking parties and gangsters'. The newspaper insisted that juvenile delinquency was 'unknown in the olden-time tribal state'. Not surprisingly, most black city residents, while embracing a Western value system, tried to cling on to some vestige of rural custom.[184]

(Left) Young male initiates outside Port Elizabeth, Eastern Cape

(Right) Paris Evangelical Mission at Seshoma, 1885

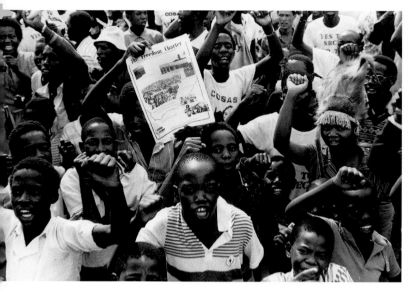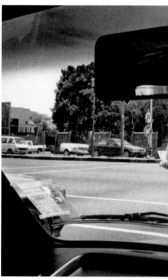

Anti-Apartheid UDF rally, 1985

New social groupings such as youth gangs and mass schooling began to take on the role of more traditional forms of sexual socialisation. In urban environments, many of the activities of male youth were unsanctioned and took place beyond parental influence. The authority of older people was questioned. Social workers expressed concern about some of the negative consequences of youth behaviour they observed on the Witwatersrand in the 1940s and 1950s.

[They] observed on the Rand a breakdown in the taboos and punishments associated with premarital sex. Fathers were not subjected to fines (as was the custom in the rural areas) or any kind of social disapproval. Increasingly, the girls' parents would accept the pregnancy after perhaps only mild rebuke.[185]

In previous decades, tradition had to some extent regulated sexuality in the urban areas through, for example, 'home-boy' networks on the mines, where young men were prevented from spending their wages on prostitutes.

The urban school environment also provided some degree of adult supervision, particularly for young girls (although girls were also subject to sexual harassment in schools). However, political youth culture, which dominated the 1970s and 1980s, had a more profound influence on their sexual behaviour. In this highly politicised environment young people learned from and taught each other and ignored the advice of elders. Increasingly they were left to their own devices as they entered adolescence. They charted their paths of sexuality amongst peers and on their own.[186]

The HIV/AIDS epidemic revealed the extent of the breakdown of parental authority and the lack of control over adolescent sexuality. Youth, in particular, were and are most at risk of infection. In the 18-to-29-year-old age cohort approximately 27% of men and 30% of women are HIV infected.[187] One of the responses to the HIV/AIDS crisis has been to look back to tradition. If AIDS is a disease associated with modernity and with the breakdown of traditional codes and prac-

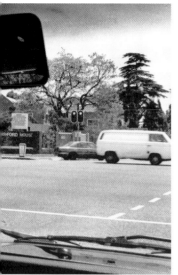
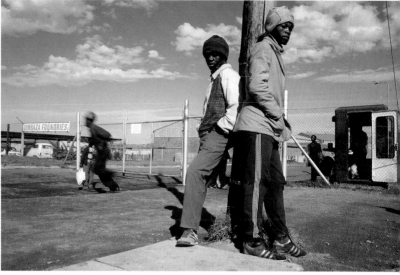

Many men and women will never find work in South Africa's formal economy

tices, then a return to traditional customs is an attempt to take control over young bodies, sexuality and reproductive health. Mass, public virginity testing in KwaZulu-Natal has been one of the most controversial attempts to reinvent tradition. Billed as an effort to promote female sexual chastity and as an AIDS-prevention strategy, the practice set traditionalists on a collision course with human rights institutions in South Africa, which claimed that virginity testing was a violation of the right to privacy.

The resurgence of virginity testing in its contemporary form is an effort both to reclaim the past and to reassert control over the future. One woman explained her support for virginity testing:

You see, our young ones … are suffering from AIDS because they don't look after themselves. They are just doing sex everywhere; now, in our culture … we Zulus, we are not allowed to sleep with a man without being married. That means we must be virgins all the time. So there are women who are doing that job, by examining them.[188]

Older women are attempting to reassert their authority over young women's sexuality by publicly testing them and imposing sanctions on those that are not virgins. Ironically, though, because of the myth that having sex with a child virgin can cure AIDS, virginity testing actually renders young women more vulnerable to rape by older men.

It is not surprising that in times of crisis people who have experienced a deliberate and systematic erosion of their cultural traditions seek to reclaim and reassert them. AIDS education and prevention campaigns have often been thwarted by the claim that 'it is not in our culture'. AIDS educators struggle to get culturally appropriate safer-sex messages across. However, far from being static, culture is constantly being re-invented in accordance with changing circumstances. The escalating rates of HIV infection are a symptom of the failure to adapt. Arresting the HIV/AIDS epidemic will require profound behavioural changes across cultures.

AIDS – AN APARTHEID ILLNESS?

AIDS cannot be described as an apartheid illness in the sense that once apartheid has finally gone AIDS will disappear too, but there is no doubt that the policies and consequences of apartheid exacerbate the spread of infection.[189]

Following the election of the National Party government in 1948 the system of migrant labour and African disenfranchisement was formalised and deepened. Apartheid served to extend the system of migrant labour indefinitely by draconian legislation and the strict control of urban migration through influx-control laws. In other industrialising countries migrancy was replaced, in time, by permanent urban settlement. But South African labour was legislated to a state of permanent mobility. Apartheid policies developed an elaborate system of social engineering including large-scale forced removals and relocation.

From the late 1950s, in pursuit of the government's policies of apartheid, South Africa was also the site of some of the most massive population movements in peacetime, outside of the Soviet Union. Over three million people were uprooted and their communities destroyed under a variety of apartheid laws.[190]

The apartheid era also saw the rapid deterioration of rural areas. Up until the 1950s, while rural communities were heavily dependent on migrant remittances they were still able to draw some support from rural production. But the intensification of influx control and the large-scale movement of people from white farms and areas defined as 'black spots' into the reserves led to a rapid rise in populations and increased pressure on land. Attempts to remodel rural communities through betterment and rehabilitation schemes further undermined their social fabric and economic viability and exacerbated the problems.

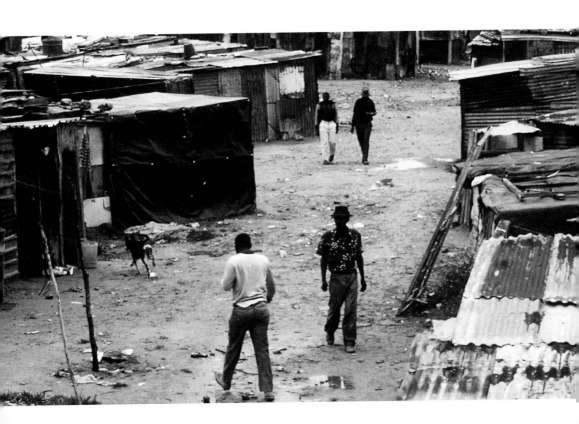

The expanding economy in the 1960s generated high levels of employment for migrants and this moderated the damage to some extent. But the steady rise of unemployment from the late 1970s had devastating consequences for many rural households, which now found themselves stripped of both rural resources and migrant remittances. The 1996 census found that 34% of the total economically active population (aged 15–60) was unemployed; the figure was 40% for Africans generally, and close on 50% in the poorest provinces.[191] According to the Poverty and Inequality Report (1998) 30% of economically active South Africans are unemployed.[192] Other studies put the figure at 35%.[193] More significantly, however, broad unemployment stands at 60% for youth below 20 compared to 12.5% for people over 55. Alarmingly, 72% of the broadly unemployed have had no prior work experience. Quite literally, this means that many men and women will never work in South Africa's formal economy and many who have been retrenched now form part of the category 'long-term unemployed'.[194]

The destabilisation of African families through migrancy, impoverishment and the destruction of communities would later contribute to the rapid spread of HIV/AIDS in the region.

Apartheid unravels

With the collapse of influx control in 1986 mushrooming squatter camps around the main towns became a prime staging post of circulatory migration. By the early 1990s it was estimated that seven million people were living in informal settlements.[195]

Given the pace and extent of urbanisation the abolition of influx control was inevitable. However, this did not lead to improved living conditions in cities. Instead, it was followed by a period of intensified violence and social dislocation.

By the mid-1980s, the combination of repressive urbanisation policies, acute housing shortages, the recession, and conditions in homelands and farming areas, all conspired to produce a wide array of shack settlements. Between 1986 and 1989 the total number of free-standing shacks in the Pretoria – Witwatersrand – Vereeniging region (PWV) increased from 28 513 to 49 179. Of the forty-seven shack settlements in early 1990, twenty-five were situated within proclaimed black townships and twenty-two were located in peri-urban areas and on land designated for white, 'coloured' or Asian residents.[196]

Informal shack settlements

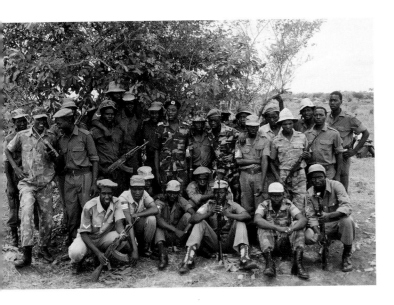
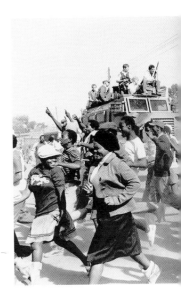

**Umkhonto weSizwe (MK)
combatants in Uganda, 1993**

Once the coercive state apparatus began to give way from the late 1970s, the huge influx of the rural impoverished and unemployed into the urban shacklands intensified the poverty and further compromised the health status of thousands of people. For rural blacks, the mode of survival represented by labour migration became so deeply entrenched that the disintegration of apartheid did not end population mobility. Instead, it actually accelerated even larger movements of deeply impoverished people into the urban areas, many of them easy prey to the diseases of poverty like malnutrition and tuberculosis, to parasitic infections and to sexually transmitted diseases. All these diseases also lower resistance to HIV infection. And the absence of social cohesion is itself a major risk factor in AIDS. It is no surprise to discover that today the more disrupted informal settlements around South Africa's cities have the highest rates of STD and HIV infection.[197]

The combination of growing unemployment (and poverty), the collapse of influx control, the increase in squatter camps and a sharp rise in political violence in the late 1980s and early 1990s led to an explosion of disease generally, for example TB. It also created an environment of social dislocation in which HIV/AIDS flourished.

How apartheid affected health

The effects of apartheid permeated every aspect of social life. Its effects on the health of the population are felt to this day. Many health-care problems are the result of apartheid policies that entrenched migrancy, enforced rural–urban drift, and led to the proliferation of squatter camps and informal settlements in towns and cities. For decades communicable diseases like gastroenteritis, measles, polio and TB were rampant and prevention and treatment programmes were wholly inadequate. These diseases were primarily located within impoverished African communities where poor water supply and sanitation exacerbated poor health status. They were virtually non-existent in affluent white suburbs. Hospitals and clinics were under-resourced, under-staffed and unable to cope with increasing demand. In 1991 the infant mortality rate (IMR) was 54 per 1000 live births. For black children the IMR was

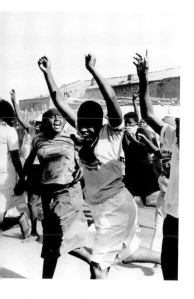

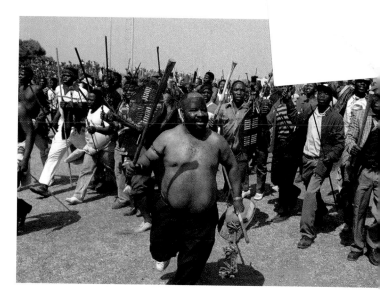

Protesters flee apartheid troops
in the townships, 1980s

Inkatha rally in Tokoza township,
East Rand

between 94 and 124 per 1000 live births. In
1989 the maternal mortality rates were 8 per
100 000 for white women and more than 58
per 100 000 for African women.

State-sponsored violence intensified in the
dying days of apartheid. A low-intensity war
waged within and beyond South Africa's
borders further unsettled communities,
especially in the conflict-ridden regions of
Gauteng and KwaZulu-Natal. War creates
the perfect conditions for the spread of
AIDS: the movement of combatants across
national borders, acts of rape and sexual violence that are associated with war, the presence of commercial sex workers and transient sexual relations.

Young 'comrades' in the townships of South
Africa often spearheaded the anti-apartheid
struggle. Sexuality was a central part of this
particular brand of urban youth culture and
regularly involved sexual subordination and
coercion of girls by comrades. The young
male comrades promoted the idea that it
was their duty to father more soldiers to
replace those who had died in the struggle

against the apartheid state. Many girls were
persuaded to abandon contraception and
those who resisted ran the risk of a severe
beating or rape.[198]

Political volatility and turbulence masked
the progress of HIV/AIDS. In the 1980s early
warning signals were either ignored or dismissed. However, the National Party government began to respond to the looming AIDS
crisis at the end of the 1980s when the
Minister of Health and Population Development, Dr Willie van Niekerk, acknowledged
that 'although a relatively small number of
cases have been diagnosed so far in South
Africa, the disease certainly has the potential to become a major problem.'[199]

You tell me AIDS can make me ill in ten years. But
twenty-five people died here last weekend. My
father died young of TB before it was called an
opportunistic infection and my brother, out of school
for three years, still has no job. Can AIDS really make
life worse than it is already?[200]

The early 1990s represented a missed opportunity for curbing the spread of HIV/AIDS. The immediate concerns of political transition overshadowed all other issues. The intangible and unseen HIV/AIDS epidemic receded in the face of immediate political considerations. Perhaps one of the greatest setbacks in curbing the spread of AIDS, especially amongst youth, was the assassination of Chris Hani in 1993. A heroic figure, Hani was poised to assume a key leadership role in the new democratic order. Unlike many other ANC leaders, he recognised that AIDS was a massive threat to political freedom. Speaking at the 1990 ANC Health Conference in Mozambique, he said: 'We cannot afford to allow the AIDS epidemic to ruin the realisation of our dreams.'

At the time of political change youth culture became much more explicitly consumerist and materialist. A number of multinational companies producing designer labels had withdrawn from South Africa because of apartheid. As this era drew to a close, local markets were flooded with goods and images selling 'the good life' to South African youth. Designer clothing, accessories and beauty products were highly sought after. The dominant image of South African youth during the apartheid period was that of resistance, captured in the image of Hector Pieterson. Post-apartheid symbols are more likely to be images of material success: designer clothes, cell phones and flashy cars.

The tragedy is that the promise of economic opportunities remains unfulfilled. Black economic empowerment has benefited only a small elite. It is no surprise that the best-resourced AIDS awareness organisation aimed at South African youth models its campaign on the advertising strategies of major international corporations. It brands its product on massive billboards throughout the country in an attempt to reach its target market.

The transition to democracy heralded an entirely new political dispensation based on the principles of human rights. Among these was the promise of improved health care for the majority of the population. Before this could be accomplished, however, government departments and the health-care system had to be restructured. This entailed incorporating fourteen apartheid-created departments of health into one national health department. More than any other area, health required far-reaching reorganisation. Health officials who had begun to notice changing patterns of morbidity and causes of death became embroiled in bureaucratic restructuring. Thus a vital moment in the progression of the epidemic was overlooked.

Prior to the 1994 elections the formation of the National AIDS Committee of South Africa (NACOSA) in 1992 and the formulation of a comprehensive AIDS programme signalled the government's intent to tackle the AIDS epidemic. NACOSA represented a coordinated national effort that straddled political differences and included the major political players of the time. When the ANC government came to power in 1994 a national structure was already in place but the government failed to take effective action based on the national AIDS plan.

Two years later a public scandal erupted when it was revealed that a government contract of R14 million had been granted to create an AIDS musical called *Sarafina II*. This generated an enormous amount of negative media attention for the government and was the subject of the first investigation by the new office of the Public Protector. President Mandela acknowledged that *Sarafina II* was one the ANC's 'three mistakes' of 1996.[201]

As the *Sarafina II* scandal was dying down government announced the development of a South African treatment for HIV/AIDS: Virodene (an organic solvent). The Medical Research Council declined applications for further testing on humans because of serious concerns about the safety of the drug and insufficient proof of its effectiveness. Ultimately, the severe toxicity of the drug was exposed and it lost credibility as a viable treatment for HIV/AIDS. The drug also embroiled the Minister of Health and then Deputy President Thabo Mbeki in a public altercation with the Medical Research Council.

In 2000 President Mbeki established an AIDS Advisory Panel that included some discredited scientists who questioned the link between HIV and AIDS. He severely tarnished his international reputation by engaging in ill-informed public debates about the causes of AIDS. He echoed the views of AIDS dissidents and still refuses to make an unambiguous statement about the causality of AIDS.

Despite the public controversy, government departments funded national AIDS education and prevention programmes. In some areas, mother-to-child-transmission pilot sites were established to make Nevirapine available to pregnant mothers.

CONCLUSION

In attempting to understand how the HIV/AIDS epidemic took root in South Africa and how it spread exponentially we have argued that the answer lies in South Africa's complex history. It was indeed an epidemic waiting to happen. Earlier epidemics show some significant parallels with AIDS. This points to the way in which economic disparities and social transitions shape the nature and pattern of disease. A key lesson to be learned from other epidemics is that they cannot be separated from the social environment in which they occur. They thrive in a context of social inequality. AIDS is no exception. However, AIDS shows some unique and distinctive features which make it more virulent and dangerous than any virus we have seen before.

CULTURAL COLLISIONS:
POPULAR UNDERSTANDINGS
OF HIV/AIDS

Popular explanations of HIV/AIDS

Understanding AIDS through the paradigm of witchcraft

Co-opting traditional healers in the fight against HIV/AIDS

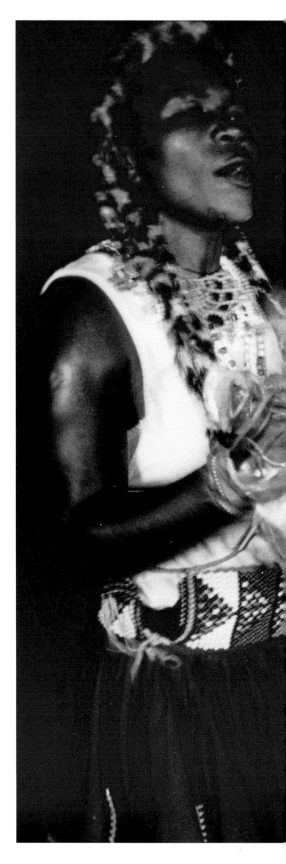

Sangoma ritual in KwaZulu-Natal

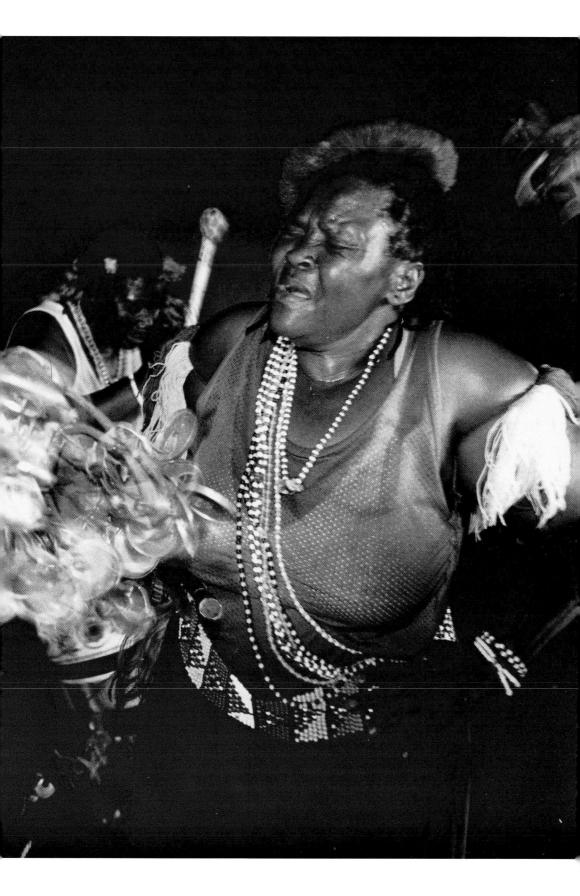

How do we understand AIDS? What causes AIDS? Why do some people become infected and others not? Questions like these are often informed and answered by our belief systems or worldviews. Our belief systems are shaped by many factors, including our cultural, religious and ethnic background, our family and personal history, our gender and our economic circumstances. These systems are learned, shared, and constantly changing, and are the means through which we interpret and generate social behaviour. They are the lens through which we view many issues, from daily tasks (such as how we dress and what we eat) to fundamental life-threatening experiences (such as disease and death).

Belief systems impact directly on how we understand health and respond to illness. They influence how we make sense of the causes of disease and help us to understand how healing takes place. Every community has well-established ways of maintaining health, preventing disease and treating the sick. Some individuals and communities understand disease to be caused by magical and spiritual forces, others draw on scientific reasoning and many apply both models. There is a range of competing explanations that can be drawn on. Symptoms that are considered 'normal' in one social context are not considered normal in another. Similarly, there are social differences in the way people respond to symptoms. Who people choose to go to when they are sick and their reactions to prescribed treatments and remedies differ from one family (or community) to another.

South African society is characterised by cultural complexity and difference. This is reflected in the many ways that health and disease are understood. There are many health-care systems in this country, each rooted in its own worldview and each with its own claims. In explaining, preventing,

Madam, please don't get angry, but did you ever think about why everybody is talking about AIDS, AIDS, AIDS? This is a European word! We healers in Africa have known about AIDS long before the British. We call it *kanyera*.[202]

treating and managing HIV/AIDS in South Africa, different cultures and belief systems have collided, often with serious consequences. For example, Western medicine diagnoses epilepsy as a neurological disorder that can be effectively managed by prescribing certain treatment. However, in some Asian cultures the symptoms of epilepsy signify a special spiritual status. It is not a condition to be treated medically.[203]

Throughout the world, the biomedical or scientific model has dominated explanations of the causes and treatment of HIV/AIDS. In this medical system the cause of the disease is a virus, and the focus of prevention and treatment the individual patient. The biomedical model lies at the heart of most AIDS research, intervention and education programmes in South Africa and internationally.

The acceptance of biomedical models of the disease has been so much to the forefront that other understandings have been subdued ... as the product of 'ignorance' or of outmoded traditional views by those primarily involved in the AIDS field, both by government personnel and Western AIDS specialists. The language of AIDS is the language of Western science and policy. All programmes in Africa, whether medical or social, have been dominated by the WHO, and more recently UNAIDS, as well as USAID and other Western-based NGOs.[204]

This has had negative repercussions on efforts to combat the epidemic in Southern Africa. Research has shown, for example, that the impact of AIDS intervention programmes in Botswana has been negligible because the model of intervention was based on Western experiences and expertise (the biomedical model). The emphasis in these programmes (as with most others in Southern Africa) was on protecting the individual, primarily through the use of condoms, as well as promoting abstinence and monogamy. It was assumed that these

Western experiences were generalisable to a range of vastly different social situations.[205]

For example, the safer-sex model of prevention was initially developed and used in the West in the 1980s. Aimed at affluent gay men, it was based on the idea that given the 'facts' and presented with alternatives, people will change their sexual practices in order to avoid HIV. It was assumed that this particular model could be imported to any part of the world and aimed at any group of people.

However, educators conducting a life-skills education programme in primary schools in KwaZulu-Natal found that it was necessary to develop a culturally sensitive approach based on aspects of 'Zulu cultural meaning systems'. This was in direct response to the (biomedical) health belief model, which the educators found unhelpful and inappropriate.

The model is based on the premise, for example, that in the light of information she is given, and her beliefs or attitudes, a woman will choose healthy behaviour. This model does not take the social circumstances in which the woman lives sufficiently into account. Personal choice is not a simple matter. She may have to choose between securing some food for herself and her children and taking a health risk by having sex with her husband who she suspects could be infected with HIV. Health-belief theories inform current national life-skills programmes [and] priority is not given to the social circumstances of the learners. Current life-skills programmes are based on Western values. They are founded in concepts such as independence, individuality, decision-making, self-concept and assertiveness.[206]

Scientific or modern medicine offers rational, measurable and directly observable explanations for disease. Illness may be linked to individual lifestyle but certainly not to spiritual forces. Remedies and cures are provided without an accompanying rationale.

However, many millions of people who consult medical doctors and nurses also defer to healers who are located within other healing systems. People living with HIV/AIDS are no exception. For example, in Botswana and South Africa, people seek advice from a combination of Western doctors, diviners, herbalists and prophets based in independent spirit churches. And traditional healers are increasingly being seen as legitimate health practitioners in South Africa. For example, some medical aid schemes reimburse members for visits to traditional healers.

A study of sex workers in Hillbrow, Johannesburg, showed that they consulted both medical doctors and traditional healers. In fact they showed no preference either way. But some did comment on the different role each played in maintaining health. 'Traditional doctors uproot the disease while biomedical doctors cure it.'[207]

There are two broad types of African healing practitioners in South Africa: faith healers and traditional healers. Both draw on a range of diverse traditions and can be further divided into subsets. In South Africa we find the *sangoma*, 'who is possessed by spirits and who has been initiated into a healing cult, and the *inyanga* (herbalist) who is simply a person knowledgeable about African medicinal herbs ... The *sangoma* is distinguished from the *inyanga* primarily by the *sangoma's* belief that he or she is possessed by one or several spirits, and by the *sangoma's* ... having experienced some life-threatening illness that has been cured through their apprenticeship to a senior *sangoma*.'[208] These are neat categories but they are not always clear-cut. The practice of traditional healing takes different forms, and *sangomas* and *inyangas* combine different elements in their work.

Training workshop in AIDS education for traditional healers. In this role-playing, a traditional healer teaches her patient about AIDS prevention.

Collaboration between traditional healers and conventional medicine

In the 1950s, the founder of the Valley Trust, Dr Halley Stott, entered into a partnership with the traditional healers in the area, which was continued by Dr Irwin Friedman in the 1980s.

The traditional healers and Western doctors have been working together in preventing and managing common diseases in the area for over 40 years now, and as a result of their successful collaboration they were recently given an award at a meeting of the *Inyangas'* Association in KwaZulu-Natal, for serving as an example to the rest of the traditional healers and Western doctors in South Africa.

Mrs Nokusho Vhengu, who graduated as a *sangoma* in 1966, was one of the first traditional healers to work in partnership with the doctors of the Valley Trust. In the 1980s,

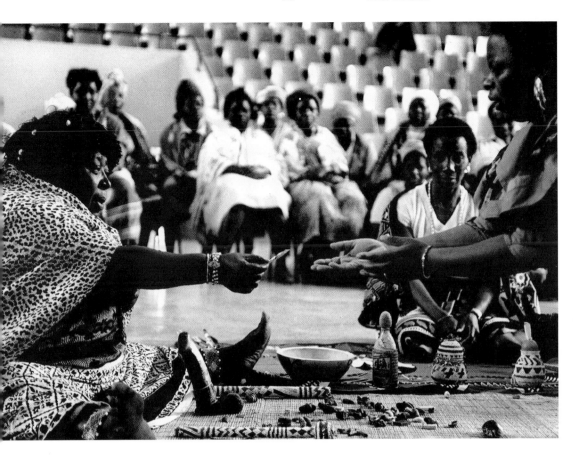

she and a number of other traditional healers and community members were trained as community health workers. The traditional healers have never seen their simultaneous practice of traditional medicine and Western-based primary health care as conflicting. In fact, Mrs Vhengu feels that all traditional healers should be given a course in primary health care before graduating.

The traditional healers working within the Valley Trust are involved in numerous aspects of primary health care. There are currently 90 traditional healers working within the framework of the Valley Trust, treating patients with traditional methods if they feel this is appropriate, or referring them to the clinic doctors if necessary. The patients report back to the traditional healers after consultation at the clinics. According to Mrs Vhengu, the patients are happy with this arrangement as they see the Western doctors as treating the

symptoms of the disease and the traditional healers as treating the cause. With this system, they perceive their treatment as complete and holistic.

Dr Friedman says, 'Traditional practitioners are an integral part of the culture of the society. Just as with other individuals they are part of dynamic social change. My experience has suggested that in many respects they are leaders of social change and are early rather than late adapters of new ideas. Traditional practitioners are enormously influential in improving people's health. My own view is that we, as Western practitioners, must come to a much closer understanding for ourselves of traditional healers as a prelude to any policy formulation. I don't believe we can define a role for traditional practitioners unless it is done in the spirit of genuine partnership.'[209]

The scope of traditional healing is reflected in the South African traditional healers' *Primary Health Care Handbook*. The traditional healer deals with the following categories of conditions:

- **Conditions of the respiratory system:**
  colds and flu; hay fever; pneumonia; asthma; bronchitis; emphysema; tuberculosis.

- **Conditions of the gastro-intestinal system:**
  diarrhoea; dysentery; constipation; heartburn; indigestion; ulcers; haemorrhoids; worms.

- **Conditions of the cardiovascular system:**
  angina; high blood pressure; palpitations.

- **Conditions of the central nervous system:**
  headache; migraine; stroke (traditional treatment is given after discharge from hospital).

- **Conditions of the skin and hair:**
  acne; eczema; boils; insect bites and stings; ringworm; scabies.

- **Conditions of the blood:**
  anaemia; blood cleansing (routinely given following treatment to help cleanse the body of the original cause of the disease).

- **Conditions of the urogenital system:**
  sexually transmitted diseases; cystitis; menstrual pain; vaginitis.

- **Conditions of the eyes:**
  'pink eye'.

- **Conditions of the musculoskeletal system:**
  arthritis; backache; muscular pain; gout; sprains and strains; rheumatism.

- **Other conditions:**
  cancer; HIV/AIDS; fever; pain; alcoholism.

There are an estimated 150 000 to 200 000 traditional healers in South Africa.[210] It is believed that as many as 80% of African people consult traditional healers and they do so for a number of reasons. The absence of hospitals and clinics in many regions (particularly in rural areas) and understaffed and overcrowded health facilities (where they do exist) partly account for widespread reliance on traditional healers in many Southern African countries. Indeed, during the apartheid years, the government often used the resort to traditional healers as an excuse not to provide health facilities. Yet even when health services are accessible, millions of people still choose to confer with traditional healers. This is because they provide a 'psychological and a physical diagnosis that relates the complaint to the social milieu of the client'.[211]

Illnesses are understood to have a social cause, be they the consequence of bad relationships or the result of some action taken by the patient (or a close relative). Traditional healers usually take a holistic approach, dealing with all aspects of the patient's life, social context and psychological state. They provide culturally familiar ways of explaining the cause and timing of ill health and its relationship to the social and supernatural worlds. Healers provide medicine for the 'affairs of daily life'.[212] They also provide a conceptual framework that helps many of their patients to understand their illnesses.

For many Africans the logic of scientific medicine is not obvious, although its effects are clear and fully accepted. The traditional healer works within a cultural framework that is familiar and understood by many Africans as both powerful

Turning to traditional healers

The rapid spread of AIDS, combined with the expense and difficulty in obtaining Western medicine, is forcing more people to consult traditional healers in search of a cure. But do the government and other players in the medical fraternity appreciate their role?

Prudence Mabele (30) is among the growing number of AIDS sufferers who believe traditional herbs have medicinal properties that could help in the search for an AIDS cure. She says that ever since she started taking traditional medicines she has regained her appetite and has even improved physically.

Why did she turn to traditional healers, whose methods of treatment were not only perceived as obscure but also unscientific? 'Because traditional healers use natural herbs which do not have side effects. They are also readily available.' She says, 'I pay as little as R50 to get traditional medicine, while I have to spend thrice the amount to get Western-based medications. Traditional herbs have sharpened my appetite and also rid my system of foreign substances.' Perhaps more importantly, 'I find traditional healers to be more genuine, humane and caring than some of the nurses in the government hospitals and clinic who display this uncaring, arrogant attitude to AIDS sufferers.' However, 'this will not preclude me from using any stuff whatsoever that has been proven to prolong life.'

Mabele says traditional healers are doing a fine job; however, they need to coalesce and work as a team so that they are a force to be reckoned with. 'This will enable them to have their own laboratories, own land to cultivate herbs, package them properly and even learn something about dosage.'[216]

and effective – if not in all cases, then in some. Moreover, the logic of the therapy for many Africans (though by no means all) is understandable and consistent with a broader worldview and concept of the person as a human being with social, physical and spiritual aspects.[213]

Unlike Western medicine, traditional medicine emphasises spiritual dimensions of the self. Its diagnosis of illness or misfortune includes a spiritual explanation. In this healing system the role of an individual's ancestors is seen as particularly important. Ancestors are the guardians of social norms and values and 'they have the power of unmediated intervention in the lives of their descendants'.[214]

Systems of modern medicine and traditional healing exist side by side, each providing a different function, and many people move back and forth from one system to another. A case study on the impact of religion on HIV/AIDS prevention and education programmes in Tanzania shows how spiritual and scientific explanations of HIV/AIDS coexist.

In these local contexts the discourses on moral and spiritual causes of the disease are often as real as the biomedical explanations themselves. There may be a very fluent relationship between different concepts of disease, which is why it is often impossible to draw a clear line between different discourses on the same disease or to classify them within a closed medical system. The fluidity of the relation between different discourses on disease may be the reason that someone who is medically treated by an NGO and who has accepted the biomedical conception of HIV does in addition to this not exclude a moral or spiritual cause for his illness.[215]

POPULAR EXPLANATIONS OF HIV/AIDS

A study of government AIDS messages in Botswana showed that local, traditional explanations for the transmission of HIV/AIDS do exist. Some of these are rooted in Tswana beliefs and indigenous medicine.[217] Others are based on Christian beliefs. For example, a bishop of St Paul's Apostolic Faith Mission of Botswana said in an interview (expressing what he believed to be a minority view):

AIDS is a punishment sent by God, as Sodom and Gomorrah. Today we have all kinds of unnatural things – homosexuality, Satanist cults who practise cannibalism, ritual murders, bestiality. Christ is the one who said that those who do such things are cursed already. Unless we discover ourselves we are a lost people. The whole country should pray to God for deliverance.[218]

He did go on to say that the church needed to work with scientific medicine, claiming that 'AIDS could be beaten by a partnership between medicine and God'.[219]

A *sangoma* from Botswana argued that AIDS was a new manifestation of an old disease that has re-emerged because people (particularly young women) have rejected or abandoned their culture or traditional practices that may have regulated their sexuality and sexual practices.

In traditional Tswana medicine we don't believe in the existence of AIDS. There is no AIDS and if it is there it is made by *makgoa* (whites) because of the many things that they recommend to be used. There are pills, injections, condoms and the coil. [The] disease of the blanket can kill; even in the past, it killed.[220]

Similarly, a prophet of a small spirit church claimed that AIDS was due to a loss of culture and contamination through exposure to modern (Western) devices such as condoms:

Gaborone, Botswana

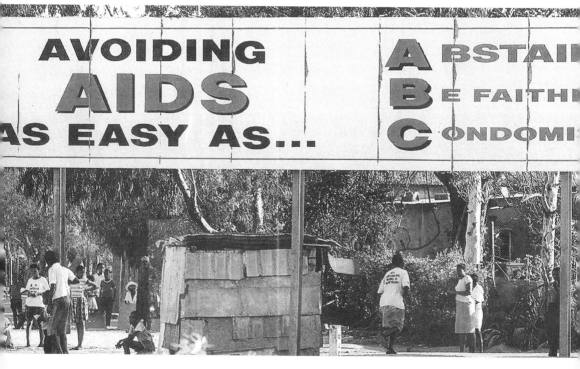

The disease of AIDS is very much related to *tonono* (result of sleeping with a woman who is menstruating). AIDS is *megare* (germs) which have been sowed in modern ways (*sesha*), but some of these germs have been there in the past, as gonorrhoea, *tonono* and *thibamo* (breech or other abnormal birth) … But for AIDS I blame the government. It has spread it. It has spread it through condoms.[221]

There are many different ideas contained in these explanations. Central is the notion that AIDS has been around for some time although in different forms. This is most apparent in the idea that inappropriate sex is potentially polluting or contaminating, resulting in a sexually transmitted disease. In Botswana for instance, STIs 'are seen to be due to the pollution incurred through breaking of sexual taboos – *melia*. These diseases are thus perversions: they link the physical and moral with "white ways" providing a reservoir of contaminating influences.'[222]

Sexual practices are regulated through a set of taboos that, if ignored or broken, will result in disease. These taboos clearly place the onus of responsibility on the woman. It is women who must not have sex during menstruation, for a period of three months after childbirth, and for a year after the death of a spouse. AIDS is blamed on the breaking of one or more of these taboos, and could indeed be blamed on women, for they are the source of pollutants. These taboos are formed through an elaborate understanding of flows of blood and body fluids between men and women. Some blood is good and other blood is bad. Appropriate flows of body fluids ensure health and physical well-being. Immediately after the death of a spouse the bereaved partner is in danger as his or her blood is said to 'stop' – to become 'hot' and 'heavy' without its partner. This may cause the bereaved partner to become ill and it poses a particular danger for any other person in sexual contact with him or her.[223]

Orange Farm informal settlement south of Johannesburg

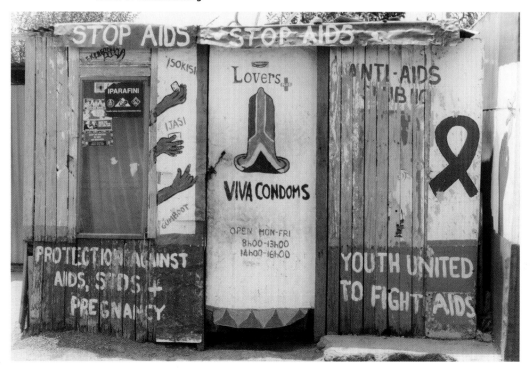

A study conducted on perceptions of AIDS among indigenous healers in Malawi uncovered a complex of diseases known as *mdulo*, which are also related to sexual misbehaviour, particularly during traditionally restricted periods. 'These diseases [*kanyera, ntayo, tsempho, malilo*] result from direct or indirect sexual contamination, from contact between defined hot and cold bodily states.'[224]

Mdulo also reflects the high premium placed on fertility and social continuity in Malawi and the need to regulate sexual conduct in order to achieve this. Amongst indigenous healers AIDS is referred to as *kanyera*, which forms part of the *mdulo* complex. Healers described how *kanyera* is transmitted:

The only way to get this disease is by sexual intercourse ... a person that sleeps with a woman who is in her monthly period (*ali ku mwezi*) can get *kanyera* ... the first thing is that ... when a woman who is in her monthly period, the man gets *kanyera*. Many people do not know that when a woman has finished her monthly period, they should wait for three days before having sex.[225]

Healers also said that a period of abstinence should be observed after childbirth. 'When she gave birth to a child, the water used to be yellow, this water is dangerous. If she has sex with a man, that blood goes to a man and then will cause *kanyera* in the man.'[226]

The symptoms of *kanyera* are very similar to HIV/AIDS, particularly those of diarrhoea, weight loss and coughing.

AIDS the sickness is not different to *kanyera*. The patients look the same; firstly they had fever (*malungo*) and they have several body pains, and next the patient feels his/her body weak. After this they start diarrhoea and then you can see through their hands. They become white

(*numayera*) and then if a person reaches this stage, then it's late with the patients, therefore it is difficult to help.[227]

Rates of *kanyera* are increasing in Malawi. According to some indigenous healers one reason for this is that young people, particularly young women, are adopting modern, Western lifestyles. Like the youth in Botswana, they are seen to be rejecting traditional cultural values and practices. AIDS is being firmly located within local cultural expectations and worldviews of traditional healers and their patients. Indigenous healers in Malawi and Botswana are using culturally familiar explanations to understand the history and origins of HIV/AIDS. STIs are seen as the result of a breakdown in the regulation of sexuality and changing sexual practices, especially amongst women. This is an example of how AIDS can provoke conservative responses that perpetuate the inferior position of women. It also raises doubts about the possibility of collaboration between Western and traditional medicine.

Traditional healers in South Africa explain HIV/AIDS in a similar way. For example, traditional birth attendants in the Free State commented on the causes of HIV/AIDS and other STIs thus:

The cause of [HIV/AIDS/STIs] is failure to comply with a traditional ritual after losing a spouse in death, post-abortion or [after] delivery. [In these circumstances] the parties are to abstain until a cleansing ceremony has been performed. A specific *muti* is drunk for a prescribed period, after which one can resume sexual relations.[228]

In this study of traditional birth attendants and their knowledge of HIV/AIDS, young people were seen to be responsible for escalating HIV infection rates because they did not abide by 'cultural or traditional prescriptions'.

A study of traditional healers' knowledge and understanding of the causes of HIV/AIDS in Gauteng and Mpumalanga demonstrated that they were well informed about bio-medical explanations of the transmission and causes of HIV/AIDS. Most healers interviewed in the study blamed HIV/AIDS on 'dirty blood' and believed that it was sexually transmitted either through sexual permissiveness or 'ritual pollution'.[229] Talking about the sexual transmission of HIV, one healer said:

AIDS is caused when two people have sex, you must not share a razor and you must always wear gloves when treating a patient. AIDS is caused by sex and not taking care of themselves, sharing of razor blades, and rubbing of two sores, that is the cause of AIDS.[230]

The idea of 'dirty blood' is an important explanatory factor for many indigenous healers. Dirt is contained in the blood and is transmitted through body fluids such as semen and vaginal fluids. 'Dirty blood is the cause of AIDS, when two people sleep together and the other party's blood is dirty, he can infect the other. It started like it was STD and then it got complicated. In fact STDs and AIDS are one and the same thing.'[231]

This 'dirt' is sometimes equated with poison. And the effects of poisoning are felt beyond the 'poisoned' individual, often impacting on an entire family or community. 'The cause of AIDS is the poison in someone's blood. We need to know how that poison gets into the body … now they say if you sleep with somebody you get AIDS, so us *sangomas*, we call it *ukufa kwendlu,* that means 'the dying of the temple' or house [body].'[232]

As in Botswana and Malawi, South African healers also see sexual intercourse in certain circumstances as contaminating. They believe that if you have sex with someone who has experienced the death of a close relative or spouse or had an abortion or miscarriage you are likely to contract an STI, known traditionally as *intsela*.[233]

Indigenous healers are not the only people who see body fluids as a potential source of contamination. A study on the perceptions of illness and disease among sex workers in Hillbrow came to similar conclusions. These sex workers defended their practice of dry sex for two reasons. Firstly, tightening their vaginas heightens their clients' (and partners') sexual pleasure; secondly, vaginal discharge is seen as a sign of sickness.

Vaginal discharge is a sign of bodily contamination, thus it is an indication of disease. Therefore they [sex workers] employ ways of keeping themselves clean and free of vaginal fluids. Women reported using agents to clean the blood and the womb. They used agents such as snuff, dry cloth, sponge, cold water etc. for drying their vaginas. They also reported using traditional *muti* (*imbiza*) and antibiotics. *Imbiza* is a mixture of herbs that is said to cleanse the blood and work as a laxative.[234]

There are many competing understandings of HIV/AIDS amongst traditional and other healers. And each has its own particular authority and authenticity. But indigenous healers do influence the ways in which health and disease are experienced and understood. For many people, they provide explanations for sickness and offer treatment and moral guidance.

Another less public, less spoken about and less researched lens through which AIDS is viewed is that of witchcraft.

UNDERSTANDING AIDS
THROUGH THE PARADIGM OF WITCHCRAFT

Many people in Africa believe in the power of witchcraft and attest to its effects on their daily lives. Witchcraft may explain misfortune, bad luck, illness and death where no other obvious reason can be found. A study of religion and perceptions of HIV/AIDS in Tanzania found that 'especially in the case of chronic or deadly illness the individual suffering is associated with spiritual forces, with witchcraft or malevolent ancestors'.[235]

Witchcraft, which can generally be understood to mean 'the manipulation by malicious individuals of powers inherent in persons, spiritual entities and substances to cause harm to others', may provide answers to the questions: why me and why now?[236] The AIDS epidemic is well suited to interpretation through the paradigm of witchcraft. It is mysterious, elusive, difficult to understand and constantly changing.

Once infected by HIV a person can remain without symptoms for ten years or more, making it difficult to pinpoint the source of infection. Moreover, the time between infection with HIV and the onset of AIDS symptoms varies widely, as does the length of time a patient might survive with the disease. Although there is widespread consensus that HIV causes AIDS, the precise mechanism by which this occurs is not well understood. Nor is it fully understood why some people exposed to the virus do not become infected.[237]

The obvious injustice of a disease that, in addition to being incurable, primarily affects the most vulnerable – the poor, the youth and the 'blameless' – fuels suspicions of witchcraft. In Soweto, Johannesburg, research shows that there are a number of popular beliefs about HIV/AIDS and witchcraft. The particular form of witchcraft to which HIV/AIDS is attributed is *isidliso* – a range of symptoms leading to a slow wasting illness. Commonly known as 'poison' or 'African poison', *isidliso* is intentionally transmitted. Often placed in food, it will harm or kill only the intended victim. Results range from bad luck (divorce, unemployment, unpopularity, family dissension) to sickness and even death. It is thus hardly surprising that *isidliso* is greatly feared.[238]

Witchcraft interpretations of HIV/AIDS can have an extremely negative impact. It has been widely reported in Mozambique and Tanzania, for example, that older women are particularly vulnerable to allegations of witchcraft when linked to the death of young people. Suspicions are aroused when young, seemingly healthy people die for no obvious reason while in the care of older relatives. Young adults who die because of AIDS and leave their children in the care of their grandparents place them at risk of accusations of witchcraft. Such allegations often result in social isolation and violence against older people.

Another negative outcome is that families who suspect that witchcraft may be the cause of illness and death have to consult traditional healers to counter the stranglehold of evil and destruction, and this can be a costly process. In order to ward off diseases such as AIDS, it may be necessary for them to pay for an extended course of treatment with a traditional healer. Typically this would be the equivalent of one month's wages for an industrial worker.[239]

The stigma associated with AIDS is often more likely to be about witchcraft than about sex. With regard to both AIDS and witchcraft silence is the norm. Just as no one wants to announce that they are cursed, few want to make their HIV status public. In the case of witchcraft, silence is part of a recognised strategy to ward off 'occult assault'.

Where HIV/AIDS is associated with witch-craft, openness about HIV status would be unlikely, if not impossible. This seriously limits efforts to de-stigmatise the disease and encourage families and communities to accept their HIV-infected members.

AIDS is seen as yet another invisible and inexplicable threat to the self and this heightens spiritual insecurity. It is particularly potent because it is incurable.

'AIDS in our midst': living with fear and stigma

AIDS is greatly feared. Popular beliefs can result in stigma and discrimination against people with the disease. In some communities the transmission of HIV is associated with the transgression of sexual taboos, health is associated with cleanliness and 'moral hygiene', and disease is seen as the outcome of forbidden exchanges and even witchcraft. It is thus hardly surprising that HIV-infected individuals are often shunned and rejected.

A study that looked at community-based care and support programmes in Gauteng and Mpophomeni found that stigmatisation, fear of HIV, and local beliefs about the causes of HIV/AIDS were the main barriers to implementing the programmes.

Metaphorically speaking, a person infected with HIV is regarded in the same light as a witch – a dangerous force that threatens the health of the community and through accusation is denied an identity as a member of that community.[240]

Family members often respond to the news that a close relative has HIV by imposing severe restrictions on their contact with other members of the household.

She [the client] complained about her sister-in-law. They gave her her own spoon, cup and a

I have seen my family die of AIDS but no one believes it

I have spent the past few months engaged in a daily struggle to 'save' the life of a man who was very close to me. This man, my cousin, was a breadwinner, a father of two who once possessed one of the strongest bodies in my extended family.

… In the end, the virus triumphed over my cousin's exhausted body. We buried him two weeks ago in Katlehong on the East Rand. He became the eighth family member I have lost to the disease over the past six years. They ranged in age from very old to the youthful. The variance in their ages and living conditions proved to me beyond doubt that nobody and no family is immune to the disease. The saddest part, however, is that with all these deaths, denial within my extended family continued and intensified.

It was not that AIDS was killing our loved ones, the dominant analysis went. It was witchcraft. Fingers were pointed at suspected neighbours and, ridiculously, even at some of my relatives. As the deaths increased, so did the list of *inyangas* who were consulted.

When I shared my concerns with my mother, she summarily silenced me and told me to keep my views to myself lest we be accused of bewitching relatives and using AIDS as our cover. This is a reaction that is common in so many families who have come into contact with the disease: denial.

As I sat watching my relative die, a nurse told me most AIDS patients that she had cared for insisted that they had been bewitched. A welfare official in KwaZulu-Natal told me that HIV-positive people arrive at her offices, holding a doctor's note recommending a social grant so they can afford nutritious foods, but still disputing the doctor's finding and arguing they have been bewitched.

Some even name those responsible …[241]

plate. She said that they [the family] give her her supper in the bedroom while the others eat in the kitchen. She also told us that her sister-in-law does not want her young child to have any food that is left over from [the client's] plate. When this happened once, the sister-in-law beat the child until she bled.[242]

This kind of behaviour has been likened to the restrictions placed on food-sharing habits and sexual contact between people and mourners to prevent 'pollution'. People with AIDS are often seen as bearers of misfortune and contamination.

In a study conducted among HIV-positive women in Gauteng it was found that all of the women interviewed kept their HIV status a secret for two to three years after being diagnosed. 'I was afraid to tell. I was diagnosed in 1995 and only told them at home this year, 1998.'[243]

For these women, the need to disclose their status arose when they or their babies became sick. For many of them the struggle to keep their HIV status a secret placed tremendous strain on their relationships – hardly surprising, as one HIV-positive woman commented: 'When I talk to people, they say all HIV-positive people should be thrown out to some place very far from the community.'[244]

Such stigmatisation and exclusion can also follow a person into death. For example, AIDS deaths in Kenya are perceived as permanent deaths.[245] If you are condemned in the world of living, then you will be condemned in the 'after-life'.

These negative responses are not limited to particular communities or groups of people. Stigmatising and rejecting people with HIV/AIDS has been a universal response, although the motivation for such reactions may be different. Some responses may be

born out of ignorance and fear; others may be explained in religious or cultural terms. Responses that arise out of popular myths may have very serious consequences. For example, there is a myth currently doing the rounds in South Africa that having sex with a virgin or an old woman can cure men of HIV/AIDS. This has led to speculation that the recent increase in child rape is a result of this myth.

Stigmatised responses to HIV/AIDS can also be traced back to the official government and medical reactions to AIDS when it was first diagnosed. Early education campaigns used scare tactics that promoted negative and stigmatising imagery.

Costing in the region of R4.5 million, the campaign [conducted by the government in the early 1990s] was aimed largely at the heterosexual population, and it was both ill-conceived and racist. Different images were selected for white and black audiences. That for whites was a fairly clichéd representation of graffiti on a wall: 'Kevin loves', the poster proclaimed, followed by many girls' names, the list of conquests crossed out and added to. Implicitly it linked AIDS to promiscuity and emphasised the benefits of a single-partner relationship. The 'black' poster showed the mourners gathered round a graveside burying an 'AIDS victim', with the caption 'AIDS kills' – linking AIDS to death. It was an extremely unpopular campaign. It dealt insensitively with the issue and took little heed of international experience, which taught that messages based on fear, judgement, doom and gloom do not work.[246]

Large-scale fear of AIDS, misinformation, popular mythology, and the legacy of mistrust left by apartheid have created an environment highly unsympathetic to those infected with HIV and living with AIDS.

First-ever AIDS awareness billboard, Queen Elizabeth Bridge, Johannesburg, 1990

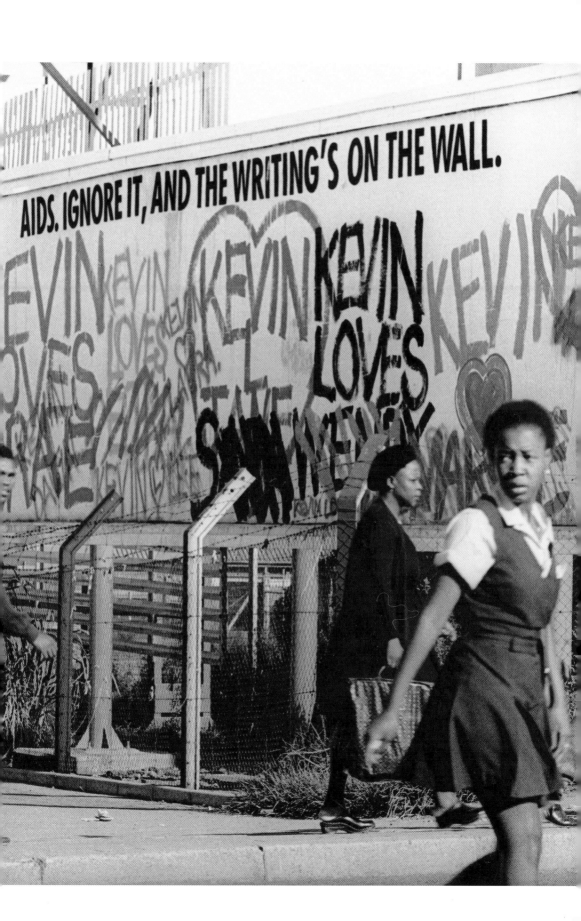

CO-OPTING TRADITIONAL HEALERS IN THE FIGHT AGAINST HIV/AIDS

The many campaigns designed to combat the spread of HIV/AIDS have largely ignored popular understandings of HIV/AIDS and the views of traditional healers. In fact, their views and practices have often been dismissed as backward, primitive and ignorant. It is true that the practice of traditional healing is alarmingly unregulated and there are many charlatans exploiting desperate people with false promises of remedies and cures. The paradigm itself is flawed because of its overwhelming reliance on spiritual, unobservable phenomena. Yet the dangers of an exclusively biomedical approach to managing the epidemic are clear.

The emphasis in all public health messages on HIV/AIDS is the practice of safe sex through using condoms. Some religious groups see this as an invitation to promiscuity. But condoms are viewed with suspicion for other reasons too. In Botswana and South Africa some people actually blame the spread of HIV/AIDS on condom use. For example, the lubricant on condoms can be seen to cause vaginal discharges – often interpreted as a sign of ill health. Also, in communities where good health is seen to depend on the appropriate exchange of body fluids, condoms are seen as a barrier to maintaining health and warding off illness.

HIV/AIDS prevention campaigns which only follow the biomedical line have messages that 'tell just one story', when there are

HIV study looks to traditional *muti*

A bold new plan involving traditional medicine in the treatment of HIV/AIDS is being explored by the Nelson R. Mandela School of Medicine in Durban. The objective of the project is to identify safe and effective therapies in the fight against the disease, looking specifically at indigenous plants used in traditional South African medicine.

Dr Ncebe Gquleni from the medical school's African Health Care Systems division said the aim was to develop a traditional system to manage the disease holistically. 'We are not only looking for substitutes for anti-retrovirals but also medicines to combat opportunistic infections associated with the disease'.

Dr Jonathan Kagan, Deputy Director of the AIDS Division at the National Institute of Allergy and Infectious Diseases, said: 'the NIH is interested in funding quality research to investigate complementary and alternative approaches to HIV/AIDS treatment and prevention.'

Sangomas and *inyangas* from Mwelela Kweliphesheya, a development arm of KwaZulu-Natal Indigenous Healers, would provide information about the flora used in traditional *muti*.

The Institute noted that 'many HIV-infected people of colour utilise complementary and alternative medicines'. Gquleni said local research supported this, with studies revealing that most people had visited a traditional healer before consulting a medical doctor.[247]

Traditional medicine being sold on the streets of Durban

other voices to be heard.[248] Indigenous knowledge systems provide an alternative way of making sense of life-threatening conditions such as HIV/AIDS. Many people think that AIDS and other STIs are the result of breaking long-standing taboos. Modern society and modern ways of behaving are also blamed for the spread of HIV/AIDS. Thus, encouraging people to adhere to traditional practices can be a way of warding off the epidemic and the modern influences that are thought to accompany it. The return to virginity testing in KwaZulu-Natal is one example of this.

While the act of refusing sex and of asserting the desire to abstain may be difficult (owing to immense peer pressure to become sexually active and to the general persistence of boys in their 'love proposals') it is also a potentially self-affirming exercise of agency. For teenage girls, faced with the challenges, rewards and dangers of impending adulthood – at a time when the very chances of arriving at that stage appear to be increasingly precarious – this act may be one of the few ways in which they are able to extend a measure of control over their lives.[249]

Many may dismiss this as a conservative backlash. But to ignore and reject the ways in which ordinary people make sense of the AIDS epidemic reinforces old divides between white and black, between Western and African, between science and magic. Stopping the spread of HIV/AIDS and treating those who are already HIV positive mean dismantling old fault-lines and developing new strategies of inclusion.

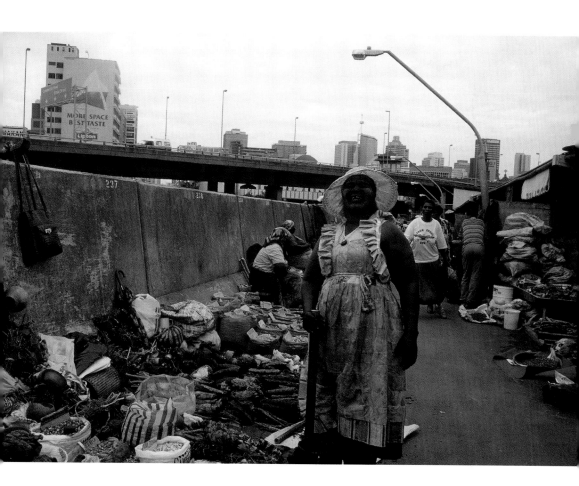

CONFRONTING THE EPIDEMIC

The legal response

Responding through prevention and care

Intervention through treatment

What is to be done?

We are burdened by a national prevalence which, when translated into percentages or absolute numbers in millions of South Africans, defies acceptance and belief.[250]

The scope and scale of the HIV/AIDS epidemic in sub-Saharan Africa is almost beyond belief. The statistics simply do not capture the human tragedy and the hugeness of the challenge facing the subcontinent. Effective intervention from states, NGOs and civil society has thus become a matter of unprecedented urgency.

Thirty-five million people in the developing world face death. Sub-Saharan Africa accounts for 70% of the world's infections and 90% of AIDS-related deaths. On average 25% of the adult population in most Southern African countries is HIV positive. Countries in the region are at various levels of maturity of the epidemic, along a north–south axis. Countries to the north of South Africa show a more mature epidemic profile. Countries further to the south, such as Botswana, Namibia, Swaziland and Lesotho, lag behind by three to four years and have experienced a rapid increase in HIV infections in the last few years. In South Africa there was a dramatic increase in HIV infection rates from 1% to 23% during the period 1990 to 1998. These high prevalence rates are testimony to the failure of interventions made by various players in the region.

The southwards gradient of the epidemic provided a 'window period' for more effective prevention strategies in South Africa. To what extent has this been a missed opportunity? What have government, civil society and the NGO sector done about the impending crisis? Which measures have been effective and which have failed? What are the current needs? How can we learn from the successes and failures of other intervention strategies? These are some of the questions that this chapter addresses.

A lot has been written about the prevention and management of epidemics such as HIV/AIDS. Medical scientists, epidemiologists and social and behavioural scientists have all contributed to an extensive body of knowledge. Here we focus on some of the ways in which the epidemic has been confronted in South Africa.

As Justice Edwin Cameron reminds us, 'our country, our region, our subcontinent, our world face an unprecedented challenge in AIDS. No other disease in history has raised, with such acute force, the ethical, political and economic questions that AIDS does.'[251]

Efforts to combat the HIV/AIDS epidemic have not resulted in smooth cooperation between different sectors of society. In fact the disease has exposed existing divisions. Government policy differs from government practice. NGOs disagree with each other and with donor agencies over effective interventions. Government is in conflict with NGOs over implementation strategies. As recent legal and political battles between the Treatment Action Campaign (TAC) and the South African government have demonstrated, civil society has been brought into direct confrontation with the state.

In the context of post-apartheid South Africa, state and non-state actors have clashed about how to define the problem, how to respond to it and who has the right to speak about it. Which civil society actors the government chooses to work with is

highly contested, as is the extent to which civil society can inform government policy.

Some analysts take this evaluation further, suggesting that struggles for access to affordable, life-saving drugs in countries such as Brazil, Thailand and South Africa have global significance. In South Africa, the TAC successfully mobilised local and international support to force several international pharmaceutical companies to back down in their bid to uphold certain patent rights. During court proceedings in Pretoria, demonstrations were taking place in the metropolitan centres of Europe and the United States.

If the rights to health and life cannot be seen to trump the right to intellectual property, the notion of rights as 'human rights' will be fundamentally undermined. One result of the HIV/AIDS crisis is that South Africa unwittingly finds itself in the vanguard of what is likely to be the first effective challenge to the neo-liberal economics rampant on the global stage since the end of the cold war.[252]

Effective AIDS activism in South Africa has challenged the worldview that justifies medical treatment for those who can afford it and a soup kitchen for those who cannot. World attention was focused on this global inequality at the Thirteenth International AIDS Conference held in Durban, 2001. It was the first time that this conference had taken place in the South. One commentator suggested that the TAC's march during the conference and Justice Edwin Cameron's speech 'forever changed the quiet acceptance of the status quo on the part of both developed and developing countries'.[253]

From blood to sweat and tears

AIDS has literally reduced well-meaning bureaucrats to weeping. Mark Gevisser suggests their frustration is part of a deeper malaise. (15 April 2001)

'Children are dying, and unnecessarily, as we speak,' said Zackie Achmat, pointing the finger at Dr Nono Simelela and Dr Helen Rees. It was at a session of the AIDS in Context conference at Johannesburg's Wits University last weekend, and Achmat, the chairman of the Treatment Action Campaign, was accusing his co-panelists of retarding the implementation of the state's mother-to-child transmission programme, which plans to administer the anti-retroviral drug, Nevirapine, to pregnant mothers with HIV.

Achmat slammed the pharmaceutical companies too: 'They regard intellectual property rights as God-given rights, and I ask, did God not give us life before he gave us intellectual property?'

But while he praised the government for its stand on compulsory licensing and reaffirmed the Treatment Action Campaign's support for the state's defence against the suit of the Pharmaceutical Manufacturers' Association (the case starts on Wednesday), he did not spare his new allies: 'We face a greater tragedy than the acts of omission of the drug companies,' he said, 'and that is the failure of government officials to act with courage, humility and urgency.'

Rees, the chairman of the Medicine Controls Council, is herself a hardened activist from the healthcare barricades of the 1980s: she responded skilfully by thanking Achmat for 'pressing our consciences' before giving her side of the story.

But when Simelela – who runs the Department of Health's AIDS programme – took the mike, her demeanour was grim and her voice shaky. It was unfair, she said, to blame her for something out of her control and in the hands of the politicians in Cabinet: 'I really have visions of being lynched by a mob, to death, for decisions that are not made by me.'

She was clearly devastated by the accusation that she had the blood of children on her hands: 'I am a mother. I am an obstetrician. The reason I chose to do this job is because of that drive and that love, and that is why I am here today ...'

At this point, in front of more than 200 politically charged academics, activists and healthcare practitioners, this soft-spoken, elegant, articulate and manifestly decent woman broke down and wept. It was one of the most awkward and uncomfortable moments I have ever witnessed.

Simelela left the auditorium as soon as she finished speaking, but Achmat was unrepentant: the Treatment Action Campaign would not be put off by tears from its mission of ensuring access to treatment for all those with HIV. 'I think this is a painful issue for all of us, because all of us watch people die, and all of us shed tears ... Pain is a thing that everyone in this room lives with, and those of us in responsible positions take it more hard, but they also have the responsibility to listen and accept criticism ... '

HIV has the eerie capacity of magnifying our social ills, of underscoring our deepest fault lines, and so it is not surprising that it has been on the stage of the AIDS epidemic that the most contentious leadership dramas of our post-apartheid society have been played out: *Sarafina II*, Virodene, the AIDS-dissident fiasco.

Perhaps this is because AIDS presents those governing this country with so profound a psychic quandary: how is it possible that, at the very moment we assume our victorious place as the leaders of a democracy we struggled for decades to bring about, we are presented with a dying populace, with a plague to which we have no answers?

'At every platform I have spoken at,' said Simelela, 'I am asked about political commitment [to fighting the AIDS epidemic]. And from my small perspective, from my very narrow perspective, political commitment is embodied in the lives of people like myself who perpetually try to communicate the constraints under which one has to work ... we are constrained by rules and regulations that are also meant to protect the very communities for which the service is meant.'

I have never met Simelela. But I would venture to guess that her tears were those of anger at being blamed for the deaths of innocent children when she feels she spends every waking hour agonising over how to save them.

I would venture to guess that they were tears of frustration, at the often-incomprehensible AIDS policy of the government; of being a civil servant caught between the rage of activists who demand action without understanding the complexities of bureaucracy and the prevarication of politicians who still do not know how to proceed.

But it seemed to me that they were tears, too, of

grief; grief for lost dreams. For as she itemised the constraints that make her job impossible, ending with the horrible ethical dilemma of having to engage in a 'calculus of misery' to decide who will live and who will die because of the scarcity of resources, I saw something I have been witnessing for a while now but have been unable to name, among both elected officials and senior bureaucrats: a sense of hopelessness and disempowerment at not being able to get things done according to the utopian blueprints with which they came to power.

These are not career politicians and career bureaucrats – well, not yet. In their hearts, many are still the activists against whom they are now pitted. They are people who have gone into the public service because of what Simelela calls 'drive and love', because of a sense of social responsibility and social justice.

They had spent their lives – in exile, in prison, in townships or on the picket lines – waiting for the moment when they could uplift their people from the iniquities of the past and prove themselves equal to the job of running a just, equitable and thriving democracy.

And now here they are, up against the wall of trying to make the grand project of post-apartheid South Africa work within the constraints of the global economy, growing unemployment, a recalcitrant and ill-trained civil service, a deeply divided society, a virus that has infected five million people and threatens to infect a lot more, and the enervating, day-in-day-out slog of running the government.

The Reconstruction and Development Programme, the New Labour Dispensation, Houses For All, Universal Primary Healthcare, Curriculum 2005: one by one the policies of redemption have had to be revised and downscaled, with their champions and drivers claiming not grand victories but small advances, pleading with the people for patience: liberation doesn't happen in a day. They are right, of course, but what are the consequences of their having come to power – and our having put them in power – believing that it did?

It is little wonder, then, that so many of them find themselves – even if they refuse to admit it – feeling disempowered.

Some respond with paralysis – they just plod into work and hope that, some day, the pile of papers on their desks will arrange itself into a pattern for redemption. Some respond defensively, with bluster and paranoia, blaming the Portuguese, the pharmaceutical companies, the media, anyone, for their inability to act according to their wishes. Some blame the iniquities of the past, and, when they do, we often respond with annoyance, not realising how profoundly disempowering it must be if you – the moral victor of the struggle against apartheid – have to perpetually blame your shortcomings on the illicit regime you thought you had conquered.

Some preoccupy themselves with the acquisition of worldly goods to assuage their feelings of powerlessness, or to console themselves that if they are not effecting profound social change, they are at least establishing the beachhead for a new middle class.

Some abuse the Marxist theory they were weaned on, to justify – more and more implausibly – the policies they are forced to implement. Many of the cleverest desert public service for the private or non-governmental sector and experience the satisfaction of something that eluded them heretofore: the pleasure of seeing the fruits of one's labour, of having agency, of making a difference, no matter how small.

What happens to those who stay? Simelela told the story of a friend of hers, a deputy minister, 'who said to me, "I slept, you people voted, I woke up the next morning and I was a minister. I didn't know what I was supposed to be doing. I had not been taught. I did not have the skills but I'm doing it, to the best of my ability."'

It is tempting to say to Simelela's friend: 'Well, if you feel you don't have the skills, give the job up to someone who does.' It is tempting to say to Simelela herself: 'If you can't take the heat, get out of the kitchen.' But that, warned another speaker on the same panel, Dr David McCoy of the Health Systems Trust, is no answer, for there is already so much dead wood in the civil service that we cannot do without people with vision, people like Simelela who are there for moral as well as professional reasons.

However, leadership requires certitude, and certitude is impossible in an atmosphere of hopelessness and alienation – even if this depression is often masked by defensive bluster and combativeness.

I saw, in the conflict between Achmat and Simelela, the public performance of the death of idealism. In our often-justified criticisms of those who run this country, we do not take the time to consider the psychic toll that their inability to act inflicts upon them, and thus inflicts upon us all.[254]

THE LEGAL RESPONSE

Human rights activists in the region have tried to ensure that laws do not discriminate against people who are HIV positive. In order to do this they work within existing legal frameworks, including national constitutions and, in the case of access to treatment, with reference to international treaties and protocols. There are advantages and limitations to the legal approach. On the one hand it is important to protect people against discrimination; on the other, the impact of the law is limited. Many face prejudice and stigma in spite of the law, which can't protect them from finger-pointing, hostility and social ostracism.

Namibia's legal framework for protection against discrimination is well developed. The Namibian Constitution asserts the principle of equality for all persons before the law and includes an anti-discrimination clause. In addition, the Constitution upholds the fundamental right to privacy, supporting other common-law legislation on privacy. This means that people have a right to informed consent before undergoing an HIV test, and the results may not be disclosed without authorisation. The Namibian government, both in terms of its own Constitution and by virtue of its status as a signatory to the International Covenant on Economic, Social and Cultural Rights, has committed itself to adequate health care for the population of the country. Labour legislation prevents employees from discriminating against anyone on the basis of HIV status. It also seeks to ensure that adequate information on AIDS is available at all places of work, confidentiality is protected and HIV-positive employees are protected from victimisation. However, 'despite the establishment of a fairly comprehensive policy and legislative framework that recognises the human rights of people living with HIV/AIDS, in practice people living with HIV/AIDS in Namibia suffer widespread rights abuses. It is obvious that good policy does not automatically translate into good practice.'[255]

The South African Constitution is internationally renowned as one of the most progressive founding documents of any nation. All international agreements that South Africa has entered into, including the Agreement on Trade-Related Aspects of Intellectual Property Rights (TRIPS), must be in accordance with the Constitution.[256] TRIPS has come into sharp focus because of its direct bearing on the ability of poorer countries to produce cheaper drugs. If interna-

The AIDS Kaffirs of Johannesburg Prison

Johannesburg inmates who have tested HIV positive are stigmatised, abused and denied rights granted to other prisoners ...

'It's like you're a snake that someone caught,' says Ben, 'a snake that everyone comes to look at.' He's struggling to find the right words to describe what it feels like to be HIV positive in a Johannesburg prison. He begins to sob as he tells how he no longer has a name, no longer has rights. 'My name is HIV or AIDS kaffir,' he says.

The Department of Correctional Services says it fully understands the serious implications of HIV infection.

A handling strategy has been circulated to prisons, and this provided for informed consent for HIV testing, counselling before and after, and confidentiality.

But prisoners tell a different story. Ben (not his real name) described in detail the manner in which he and 37 other prisoners with HIV are allegedly stigmatised, verbally and physically abused and denied rights granted to other prisoners. They were moved last month from their communal cells into isolation cells. They allege they were beaten and tear-gassed on the night of 14 June and herded into single cells. There they sit alone, unable to work or mingle with other prisoners, spending only three hours together

tional agreements are only legally binding in South Africa if they are consistent with the provisions of the Constitution, then this will affect the way in which TRIPS is interpreted in South Africa. In other words TRIPS must be compatible with the South African Constitution.

For example, TRIPS allows for developing countries to take steps to ensure that essential drugs that would otherwise be unaffordable are available. This includes the issuing of compulsory licences that authorise the use of a patent without the patent-holder's permission. TRIPS outlines the specific circumstances in which these controlled exceptions to patent law may be made. So the role of TRIPS is to balance competing interests in a way that recognises social and economic welfare. The agreement provides the broad framework within which countries may operate.

In terms of the South African Constitution the state is obliged to be proactive in ensuring social and economic as well as civil and political rights. The Constitution provides the legal basis for interpreting the TRIPS agreement. South Africa's legal framework is strongly weighted in favour of access to treatment. This has been the basis of several

court cases. In one case civil society and government were allied against international pharmaceutical companies. Other cases have been head-on confrontations between government and AIDS activists. For example, in August 2001 the TAC lodged court papers against the Minister of Health for failing to adequately implement a programme aimed at preventing mother-to-child transmission of HIV.

Civil society's response to HIV/AIDS in South Africa has a strong human rights element. Local struggles around HIV/AIDS draw on different forms of social activism. Some of these can be traced to community action in the West, notably the actions of human rights groups in the United States. Groups like ACT-UP engage in militant direct action and have a strong focus on distributing accessible information to people affected by HIV/AIDS. ACT-UP also started a new dialogue between civil society, the pharmaceutical industry and medical regulatory authorities, when it won the right to fast-track treatment while drug trials were still in progress. This form of political action has influenced local activism.

Initially local activism was directed at the pharmaceutical companies. The TAC, for

---

each day. Ben tells how the prisoners cough and cough in their cold, damp cells. 'You can squeeze the water out of our mattresses,' he says. No one comes to counsel them. If they want to get to the prison hospital in time to see the doctor, they must bribe the warden with R2 'taxi money' to open their doors early, they allege.

After visiting a doctor last year to treat the sores on his face, Ben was tested for HIV, although he claims he was not told this. A woman doctor broke the news that he was HIV positive in front of a queue of prisoners. 'The way she told me it seemed like a joke. Half of the prisoners heard what she said.'

He describes how a recently diagnosed prisoner tried to fling himself down three flights of stairs. Their food is labelled 'HIV' and when they go to collect it, everyone sees. Ben believes his illness is common knowledge in his home township. This is because the section where they are kept is across the way from the awaiting-trial section. If granted bail, these prisoners are back on the streets, spreading the news.

Asked to comment, the Department of Correctional Services said the prisoners are detained 'in a separate section of the prison to better facilitate their treatment'.[257]

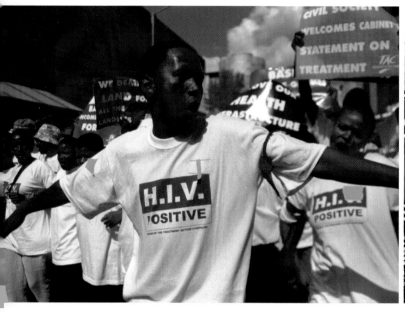

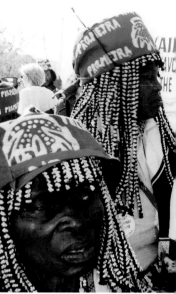

AIDS activists show support for the TAC in the Constitutional Court case to have Nevirapine supplied to pregnant mothers and children

Traditional healers gather outside the International AIDS conference venue in Durban to demand recognition for the role of traditional medicine in the fight against HIV/AIDS, July 2000

example, was set up for this purpose. The TAC also worked with the National Department of Health in the campaign for cheaper drugs. Unexpectedly, however, AIDS activist groups did not receive political support from the government and this set them on a collision course. The TAC also drew heavily on a more potent tradition within South African society – the struggle for political equality and social justice embodied in the anti-apartheid movement. In time the TAC and the Congress of South African Trade Unions (COSATU) formed an alliance around access to treatment. The TAC also supported COSATU in its campaign for a basic income grant: 'in a context of poverty and inequality, AIDS rights activism cannot escape questions of broader social and economic rights, demands which may sit uneasily with the economic and political elites.'[258]

Thus South African HIV/AIDS politics is strongly influenced by a human rights tradition, drawing on both Western and local models. This approach embodies respect for the rights of individuals, privacy and confidentiality. The rationale is that it fosters a climate of trust and tolerance, rather than one of stigma and fear. Individuals are also more likely to go for testing and to seek treatment. Thus the protection of human rights is not only a safeguard of human dignity, but also a vital ingredient in the prevention and containment of HIV infection.

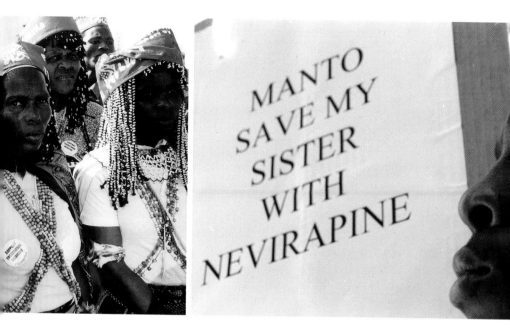

The TAC celebrates the outcome of the Constitutional Court judgment which stipulated that the government must provide Nevirapine to pregnant women and their babies

Not all health officials support this human-rights-based intervention strategy in South Africa. For example, some health officials regard the right to privacy, a cornerstone of the HIV/AIDS strategy, as counterproductive. There have been several requests by people working in the health sector and by government to limit patient confidentiality and make AIDS a notifiable disease. For example, in 1997 the South African Minister of Health unexpectedly announced that AIDS was to be made notifiable. In doing so she went against the advice of activists and scientists in the AIDS field, including epidemiologists, clinicians, NGOs and the government's own AIDS Advisory Committee. Although the minister backed down, she does have supporters within the health sector. In a recent anonymous survey of 82 senior health officials in South Africa, 70% agreed with the statement 'confidentiality is harming efforts to prevent the spread of HIV'.[259] This is part of a long-standing debate within the health profession about whether to uphold individual rights and freedoms or go with older public health responses advocating containment and control.

The legal framework is important in determining policy and ensuring that individual rights are protected. It is also an essential component of an enabling environment in which HIV infection can be prevented and contained. Good laws and policies do not guarantee non-discrimination, though; neither do they ensure access to vital medicines.

RESPONDING THROUGH PREVENTION AND CARE

Given the vast inequalities and the lack of material resources in developing countries, a number of prevention and care strategies have been tried. Peer education and community-based care are two phrases that are immediately associated with HIV/AIDS intervention work in South Africa. Both are seen to be integrated within local communities, sensitive to local conditions and, above all, affordable. However, their effectiveness is doubtful.

The origins of peer education in the HIV/AIDS sector are to be found in research related to fertility and reproductive health conducted in South Africa, notably by the Planned Parenthood Association of South

Africa. This model was adopted for HIV/AIDS prevention work. A case study of the model in KwaZulu-Natal questions some of the assumptions made by peer-education programmes. Initial attempts to introduce life-skills training through schools in the province failed. Peer education through NGO networks was then introduced. It was seen as a solution to getting safer-sex messages across to the most vulnerable sector of the population – sexually active youth.

A key element of effective peer education is 'trust'. The idea is that adolescents are more likely to trust their peers and talk about sex with them than with parents or elders. A group of young people are trained and equipped with knowledge about sexual behaviour, STIs, safer-sex practices and con-

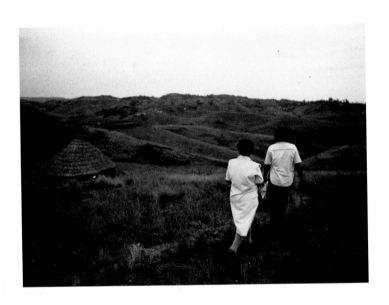

(Left) Travelling hospice in the rural districts of KwaZulu-Natal

(Right) Members of the Khutsong Youth Friendly Service hand out AIDS information in the Khutsong informal settlement, 2000

traception: information that they then share with their peers. However, the social context in which peer education takes place may work against this basic assumption of trust. Poverty and gender-based inequalities may be so pronounced that they overshadow the potential of peer education. In other words peer education may not be able to produce significant behavioural changes in an environment where there are other pressing priorities and glaring inequalities.

In some instances, peer education may reproduce these inequalities. For example, young men equipped with specialist knowledge of contraception may use their position as 'experts' to their sexual advantage. Some educators in the field acknowledged these unintended consequences.

Talking about sex

Government departments and NGOs have focused on public health prevention programmes such as massive AIDS awareness campaigns, sex education in schools, and widespread distribution of condoms. Matters of sex and sexuality have been in the public domain as never before. Newspaper articles, billboards, radio and television advertisements give both veiled and explicit sexual information. This has extended beyond the AIDS epidemic to generating public discussion of other sexual health problems such as erectile dysfunction – 'Have you taken your erection for coffee lately?' is the script of a recent radio advert.

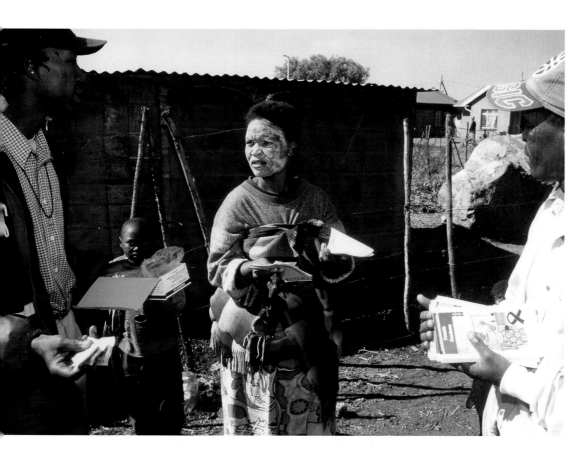

Boys will talk to girls about sex anyway, they will give out wrong information anyway – by mistake or on purpose – and they will use this misinformation to get girls to sleep with them anyway. We can only hope, with our interventions in peer education, that there will be some peer educators, among the many doing this informally anyway, and without any training, who will genuinely help. It is of course inevitable, as well, that there will be a dilution and distortion of the message. People will tell others only part of what we told them, forgetting that before this we said something very important like 'what would happen if' ...[260]

Abuse of trust, breaches of confidentiality and the coercive way in which some peer educators behave are all factors that may limit the effectiveness of this model. 'The egalitarian cosiness associated with peer education in an ideal context must surely be more frequently experienced as the duress of peer pressure in a less-than-ideal context.'[261]

Few impact studies assess the value of existing peer-education strategies. Despite this, public health officials, NGOs and donor agencies regard peer education as one of the most important interventions amongst young people.

It is difficult to weigh the positive attributes of peer education against its potential disadvantages. The difficulty is exacerbated by the fact that, because of the dearth of research, there are very few detailed evaluations of these programmes. There is a particular absence of information on the means by which, and the effectiveness with which, the programmes change sexual behaviour.[262]

In both peer education and community care programmes, public health practitioners have tended to homogenise groups and communities. In other words 'youth' are seen as an undifferentiated category of people – a particular 'target group' with relatively similar experiences and attitudes.

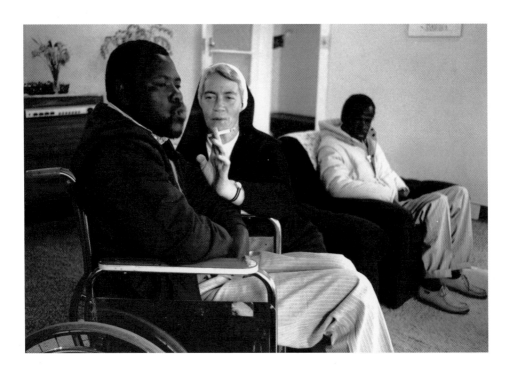

The problem is that we are targeting the general population, not specific groups. It's 'youth in South Africa' – it's a one-message-fits-all approach. We need to look more at specific target groupings. Since we cannot reach everybody, we need to look at messages for specific groups. We need to latch onto what makes a particular segment of society special.[263]

Researchers working with HIV-prevalence data echo this view. They caution against simple extrapolations that tend to see 'youth' as a single category without taking into account significant variations in behaviour and vulnerability to HIV infection.

In our recent studies of youth, it is clear that not all youth, or even young adults, are sexually active, and significant proportions of this group consistently use condoms. Extrapolating from the assumption that the general age-range population is as equally at risk as first-time pregnant women attending antenatal clinics, is an indication that the social milieu is not well understood or referenced.[264]

Community-based care has been promoted as the only viable form of care available in sub-Saharan Africa, where public health facilities are at best inadequate and at worst unavailable. Again, there is a lack of research into the actual circumstances of households and communities and their capacity to provide care. It is important to focus research attention on care provision. AIDS has a devastating effect on the economy of the household. The costs of caring for someone who is chronically ill are high. Scarce resources are used up in taking care of the ill at the expense of other pressing needs, such as food and schooling. This worsens levels of poverty and places an unbearable strain on the household.

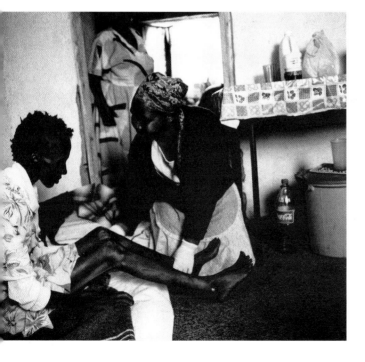

(Left) Sacred Heart AIDS Hospice

(Right) Home-based care

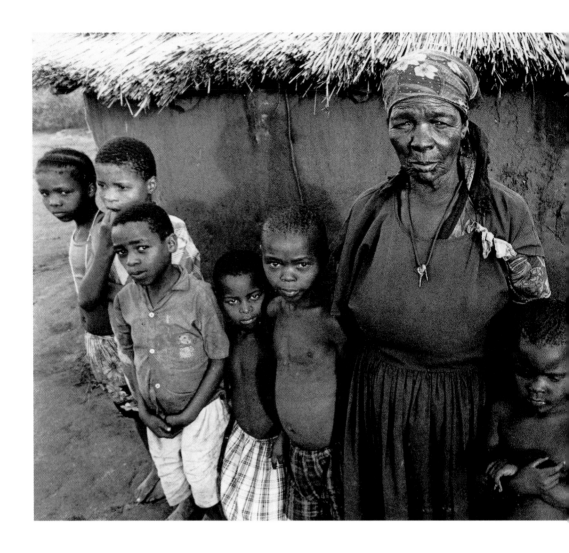

**Extract from *HIV/AIDS and the Aged*
Briefing Document**

HIV/AIDS places an already economically vulnerable group at greater risk. This is for a number of reasons. The length of time between infection with HIV and death is (in case of the adults) approximately eight years. This period is characterised by bouts of illness and good health (as with many chronic conditions). The cost of medication for treating short-term opportunistic infections is often high and money earmarked for other purposes such as schooling and household running costs is spent on this. Anti-retroviral therapy, where it is not provided free by the state, is out of the financial reach of the vast majority of people in South Africa (and beyond),

although it would reduce the cost of treating opportunistic infections as they would occur with much less frequency. This cost is often met by the older members of the family. Research in Africa (including South Africa) and Thailand has shown that HIV-infected children rely on their older parents to support them (and their children) when they are ill. If they have not been living at their family home prior to infection they often return (or move close by) when they become ill. The financial costs of the disease thus become 'family costs', which may be borne by older members of the family.

Food costs often increase. Older parents try to provide their HIV-infected children with more nutritious food in an attempt

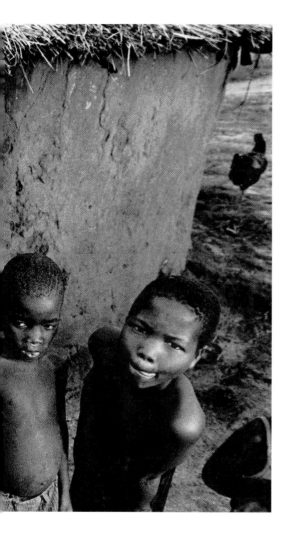

A grandmother is left to take care of AIDS-orphaned children in her village

to boost their immune systems and stave off opportunistic infections. Research also reveals that parents use food as a means of comforting and reassuring their children, for example, buying meat when they might previously not have done so because the cost was prohibitive. Healthy eating can thus be expensive eating.

Funeral costs are high and burial societies throughout Africa are under great pressure and in some cases have collapsed ... Financial and social support previously met through these informal networks are under pressure and consequently unreliable.

Costs of caring for grandchildren may also fall to the grandparents. In addition to daily living costs, this also includes schooling in the case of AIDS orphans. Grandparents may also have to cover the medical expenses of HIV-positive grandchildren if they outlive their parents.

The absence of income from the family member who is dying of HIV/AIDS (on which older members previously relied) causes long-term financial strain. The older member of the family (most often the grandmother) is required to provide full-time care and therefore cannot work. Assets may be sold to cover these costs. This loss of income compromises the entire family network.[265]

While peer education is aimed at preventing HIV transmission, community-based care tries to provide maximum support to those with AIDS-related illnesses who have limited access to facilities and resources. The problem is that most HIV-infected people in South Africa do not have access to adequate health-care facilities. And AIDS has aggravated this situation. Hospitals and hospices in the formal health-care system are increasingly unable to deal with the numbers of people who are ill or dying of AIDS-related illnesses. The state would require an enormous outlay of capital and resources and a dramatic expansion of existing facilities if it were to take on this responsibility.

Welfare organisations are struggling to cope with the growing numbers of children who are HIV positive or who have been orphaned by AIDS. By 2004 an estimated two and a half million children will be AIDS orphans. Approximately one-third of these will be HIV positive.[266]

Community-based care relies on volunteers to provide emotional and practical support to households that are providing palliative care to sick and dying relatives. The programme of community-based care is premised on several assumptions. It assumes high levels of acceptance and low levels of stigma directed at those who are HIV positive or sick from AIDS. It assumes that households are able to provide basic support and resources to the ill under their care. It also depends on the support of members of the local community who are willing to work as volunteers. However, it is not easy to ask people who are living in desperate poverty to work for free, especially when there is a perception that there are well-resourced AIDS-prevention programmes operating in the area. In spite of this, though, many volunteers value the skills that they acquire through volunteer work.

Community-based care programmes shift the burden of responsibility from hospices, hospitals, welfare organisations and other state institutions to poorly equipped and under-resourced community organisations and households that are unable to cope. These programmes have limited scope and capacity to do the work and are often unsustainable. There is also a concern about the quality of care that patients receive. Do community-based organisations have sufficient volunteers and practical resources to fulfil their role as care-providers? Are there sufficient resources to monitor the volunteers and the quality and regularity of the care they provide?

There is insufficient research documenting or analysing the impact and effectiveness of community-based care programmes. A recent study conducted in two sites – one in the village of Mpophomeni in KwaZulu-Natal and the other in Alexandra township, Gauteng – suggests that many of the assumptions about the social and cultural context in which these programmes operate are inaccurate and invalid.[267]

Households and extended family structures have been eroded over many years by large-scale social and economic processes. Rapid industrialisation and urbanisation, politically motivated migration and forced removals, the shrinking of the rural economy and the growth of migrant labour have all had a profound impact on the integrity and resilience of the household. Widespread unemployment has made the situation even worse. Many older men and women who have been retrenched will never be employed in the formal economy again. And many school-leavers have never had a job in their lives. In other words, many households were already stretched to breaking point at the outset of the epidemic. HIV infection and related illnesses have also had a profound social and economic impact on households. Many young, economically active household members have succumbed to AIDS-related illnesses, leaving behind orphaned children to be cared for by ageing grandparents. Households often do not have the resources or extended family networks required for home-based care.

These practical considerations are compounded by the stigma attached to AIDS and to HIV-positive people in some communities. A number of volunteers described the extraordinary lengths that people will go to in order to keep their HIV status a secret, even from members of their immediate families.[268]

In cases where family members do know, that knowledge often elicits a hostile response. HIV-positive people have reported a number of negative experiences at the household level, including being relieved of household duties, being isolated, being allocated separate crockery and cutlery and having restrictions placed on levels of intimacy with other household members, such as physical contact with children. Several women reported being rejected by their partners or lovers.

Negative experiences at the household level are also apparent at a community level. Early health warnings associating the epidemic with sexual permissiveness and deviant behaviour stigmatised AIDS. The commercial media also stigmatised AIDS and this has fuelled fears about the illness in the popular imagination.

The large-scale fear of AIDS created an environment unsympathetic to those already infected and had a significant impact on attitudes. Interviews conducted with volunteers and 'community members' revealed that the forced removal of people infected with HIV from the township to a special 'camp' was a fairly popular option. This gained popularity in Mpophomeni

A research project that seeks to measure the impact of micro-financing on women's empowerment has been devised by the Health Systems Development Unit of the Department of Community Health, University of the Witwatersrand, and is being tested in the South Africa's rural Limpopo Province. The following outputs are expected:

- Greater understanding regarding the links between poverty, gender-based inequalities (including gender-based violence) and vulnerability to HIV infection.

- New opportunities and tools for targeting and extending HIV education and gender awareness to the most disadvantaged members of the community.

- New evidence documenting the social and health impacts of the expanded micro-credit programme – particularly pertaining to social empowerment of participants, changes in social capital and social networks, and vulnerability to gender-based violence and HIV.

- An expanded operational model for the implementation of micro-credit and other poverty-alleviation and empowerment strategies in the context of countries with a high HIV prevalence.

- An evidence-based rationale for governments to develop inter-sectoral policies linking poverty alleviation strategies to HIV/AIDS-control programmes.[269]

following a report on national television about the growing numbers of orphans in the township. Local residents claimed that the programme had destroyed the marriage prospects of young men and women from Mpophomeni.[270]

In fact, for many HIV-positive individuals living in both Mpophomeni and Alexandra, 'community' was not an inclusive, supportive environment, but a site of exclusion and ostracism. Volunteers in Mpophomeni reported that terminally ill people were hidden under blankets in their houses in order to keep them out of the public eye. Of course, stigma has a profound impact on the efficacy of community-based care programmes. Regular visits from a volunteer may raise suspicions that someone in the household is suffering from an AIDS-related illness. Meetings facilitated by a community-based care programme in Mpophomeni had to be held secretly and under cover of darkness for fear of community reprisals.

Peer education and community-based intervention strategies have had limited success. Small-scale economic intervention has been seen as another possible strategy. A study which is currently being conducted looks at the effects of economic empowerment of women at a micro-level. Its hypothesis is that economically independent women in rural areas are less vulnerable and better placed to make independent (and safer) sexual choices than women who are dependent on men for their livelihood.[271] This long-term study will try to understand the economic underpinnings of gender inequality and vulnerability to HIV infection. It will also try to provide evidence on the effects of small-scale financial intervention at a local level.

Public health wisdom suggests that the health of a population will improve when underlying conditions of poverty and inequality are addressed. In other words, 'the health of any individual is best ensured by maintaining or improving the health of the entire community.'[272] This model emphasises social factors as determinants of behaviour. Resource-poor environments can dramatically limit personal empowerment and the ability to make safer sexual choices. If social conditions are improved, safer-sex practices will follow.

The health crisis in the region requires a range of different interventions, both imme-

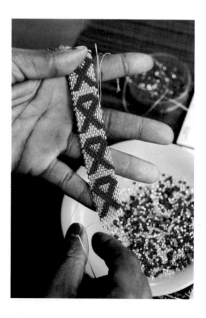

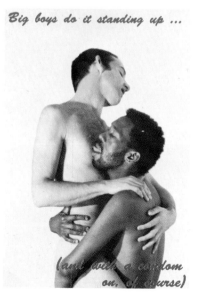

Big boys do it standing up ...

(and with a condom on, of course)

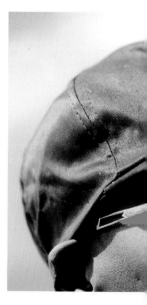

diate and long-term. Access to accurate information and preventive technologies such as condoms are essential interventions for public health practitioners. It is also essential to develop a holistic understanding of the disease in the context of sub-Saharan Africa.

Prevention and care strategies, such as peer education and home-based care, are often seen in isolation from treatment. This creates false divisions. 'Providing people with HAART (Highly Active Anti-Retroviral Therapy) helps reduce the spread of HIV. The availability of life-prolonging treatment gives people the courage to come forward and be tested and counselled, thus increasing the level of awareness about safe sex. Also, those on HAART have lower viral loads and are less infectious.'[273] Physiologically, treatment is an effective form of prevention, as evidenced by the effective prevention of HIV transmission from mother to child through the provision of Nevirapine. We argue that prevention, care and treatment are integrally connected. In short, 'AIDS treatment programmes are also AIDS prevention programmes.'[274]

Within social and health policy there has been a debate for many years about whether a person-based or place-based focus is more appropriate. I want to argue that strategies designed to reduce inequalities in health should take into account both places and people. Where people live, as well as who they are, shapes patterns of health and inequalities in health. By focusing on places we become more aware of structured differences between different types of place and the opportunities provided by the physical and social environment for people to lead healthy lives. By focusing on people, and their biographies and perceptions, we become more aware of the role of agency, power and culture in shaping how people use or fail to use local opportunity structures.[275]

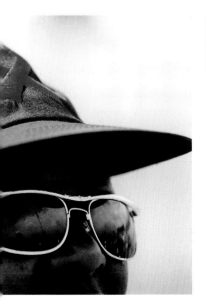

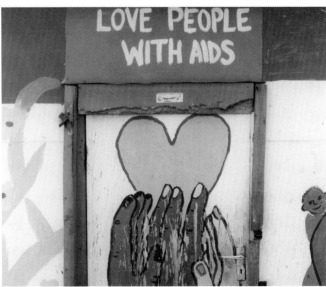

INTERVENTION THROUGH TREATMENT

The most critical breakthrough in the fight against HIV/AIDS in recent years has been the development of anti-retroviral treatment.

AIDS is no longer, does no longer have to be, a fatal illness. Life-saving combinations of anti-retroviral drugs have shown that the disease can be contained within the human body. They appear to indicate that the virus can be kept totally in check, and that under the right conditions HIV infection can be a chronically manage-able infection.[276]

Anti-retroviral drugs have changed the face of HIV in countries where they are widely available. In these countries, HIV infection is regarded as a chronic rather than a fatal condition. In South Africa this form of treatment is only available to those who can afford it. This means that treatment is currently unavailable to the vast majority of HIV-positive people.

When President Thabo Mbeki questioned the link between HIV and AIDS in 2000, he catapulted himself and his government into controversy and set the state on a collision course with HIV/AIDS activists. The Ministry of Health has taken a curiously ambivalent approach to treatment. At one point the TAC and the Minister of Health stood side by side in a court case against the Pharmaceutical Manufacturers' Association in a successful bid to win the right to produce generic drugs locally. Yet the TAC and the government appear more frequently on opposite sides in court battles.

The policies of the South African government have become one of the major obstacles to an effective treatment programme

Chronology of policy contestations on AIDS since 1994 [277]

1996	*Sarafina II* musical criticised
1997	Virodene announced
1997	AIDS made notifiable by the Minister of Health
1998-9	AZT questioned
2000	Launch of National AIDS Council by the government, excluding activists and scientists
2000	Cause of AIDS questioned by the presidency; Durban Declaration by scientists
2001	Use of ARVs in the public sector rejected by the Ministry of Health
2001	Delays in implementation of MTCT programmes by the Ministry of Health
2001	Mortality statistics questioned by the presidency

in South Africa. Other countries in sub-Saharan Africa, such as Uganda, Botswana, Namibia and Mozambique, have taken a different course, by making a commitment to providing anti-retroviral drugs within the limits of the public health-care sector. In August 2003 the South African government agreed to embark on a treatment programme. AIDS activists and the post-apartheid government have a long history of conflict, dating from public criticism that was sparked by heavy state expenditure on the *Sarafina II* musical in 1996, to the President's questioning of AIDS-related mortality statistics released by the Medical Research Council in 2001.

However, the state is not a unified entity and public rhetoric is often contrasted with actual practice. Public health practitioners are able to exercise a degree of independence while operating within state structures.

For instance, even after the [...]
questioned the link betweer [...]
the government continued t [...]
doms and buy medicines to [...]
sums of money continued to be spent o...
public health awareness campaigns based on the understanding that HIV causes AIDS, the need for behaviour change and the role of STIs as a co-factor, and condoms as an effective barrier to HIV infection.

The catapulting of AIDS into the arena of high politics has undoubtedly undermined the ability of the state to mobilise and lead a united response to AIDS in South Africa. However, conflict has tended to occur largely in the political domain and at a national level, involving mainly the presidency and the Health Ministry, with the day-to-day bureaucratic realm and provincial governments functioning relatively autonomously and sometimes in contradiction to central political stances.[278]

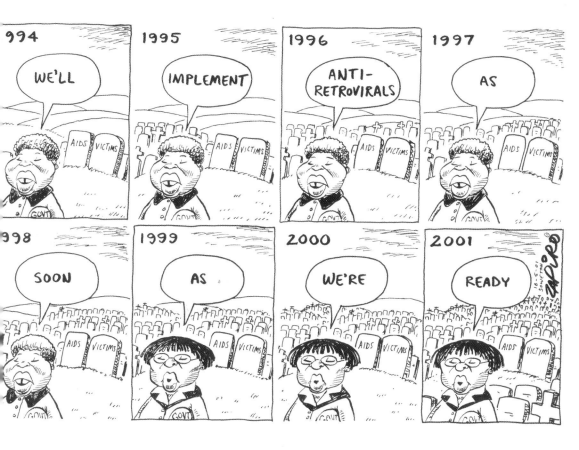

ical controversy has hindered the development of an effective treatment programme, wasting critical time in the fight against HIV/AIDS.

The South African government's stance and the absence of an HIV/AIDS treatment plan led to the emergence of a unique civil society movement. Zackie Achmat and a group of fellow activists founded the Treatment Action Campaign in 1998. The cost of medicines is at the heart of debates about treatment. In 2000 the cost of a comprehensive HAART treatment programme per person per month was in the region of R4000 (about $400). In 2003 this figure had been reduced to R1000 (about $100) per month. Importing generic drugs could dramatically reduce this cost. One estimate is that universal access to ARVs at the height of the pandemic in 2015 will cost 1.7% of GNP.

Is this a lot or a little? According to the World Health Organisation's Commission on macroeconomics and health, 'it is feasible, on average for low and middle-income countries to increase budgetary outlays for health by 1% of GNP by 2007 and 2% of GNP by 2015.' Our cost projections are within this envelope. It is not macroeconomic madness to suggest that South Africa address the AIDS pandemic by introducing a full menu of prevention and treatment programmes.[279]

South Africa would be looking at an increase of roughly 50% in national health-care expenditure. In addition to treating those who have AIDS, making such a large investment must improve the capacity of the health-care system as a whole. The cost of the drugs is not an insurmountable obstacle. The decision not to provide them is a social and political one, rather than economic.

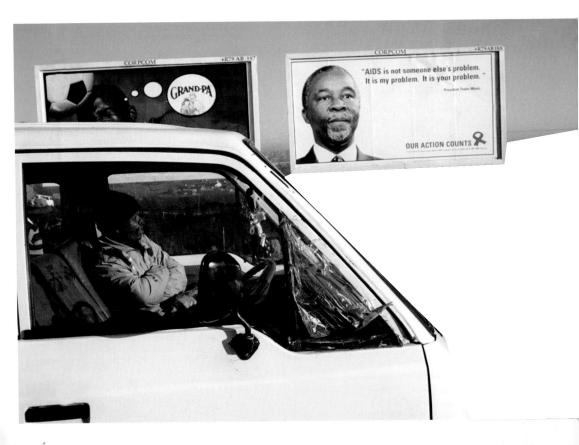

A recent study by the Centre for Actuarial Research (CARE) investigated the likely effects of various treatment and prevention interventions on the AIDS epidemic in South Africa. The results suggested that a comprehensive treatment and prevention plan was affordable and would save millions of lives. As a middle-income country South Africa can afford to provide AIDS treatment. For example, in 1999 a controversial government arms deal cost the South African taxpayer about R6.8bn.

Treatment is also important in counteracting the stigma associated with HIV/AIDS. The equation between AIDS and death is central to social stigmas and phobias. The availability of treatment would sever the link between AIDS and death and begin to undo the fear and shame that prevent open discussion of the disease. 'By preventing through treatment we give all people affected by the epidemic hope. And when hope returns to this epidemic the ignorance, fear and hatred will begin to subside. So, by showing hope through treatment, we will also address the stigma that surrounds the disease.'[280]

But offering treatment poses immense challenges. Ensuring that nearly five million people take drugs rigidly every day for the rest of their lives means confronting poverty, the hopelessly inadequate health-care service and the ongoing problems of adhering to the strict drug regimes necessary for managing chronic disease.

South Africa's health-care system manages chronic diseases very poorly. This is due as much to the lack of a trusting relationship between health-care providers and users as

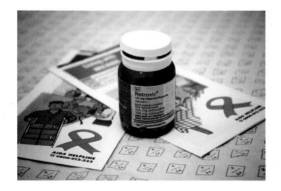

(Left) AIDS billboard in Soweto

**Government can avoid
three million AIDS deaths**
(27 September 2002)

Three million AIDS deaths would
be avoided and more than 2.5 million new HIV infections prevented
by 2015 if government provided
anti-retroviral medicines to all who
need them, new research released
yesterday by the TAC shows. The
TAC has used the research, conducted by CARE at the University
of Cape Town, to put a price tag
on providing generic versions of
the drugs in the public sector,
pointing out that the costs are
within the limits of the fiscus:
R224m last year, R6.8bn in 2007
and R18.1bn by 2015.

The findings add to growing pressure on government to change its
policy on the provision of anti-
retroviral medicines in the public
sector. One of the reasons it has
previously given for limiting the
drugs to victims of sexual assault
and occupational injury is that
they are too expensive to be made
available to everyone who needs
them. The research shows that
providing anti-retrovirals as part of
a comprehensive prevention and
treatment programme would
reduce the projected number of
children orphaned by AIDS in 2015
from two million to one million.
'This research demonstrated that,
without a comprehensive treatment plan South Africa will face a
catastrophe,' said TAC secretary
Zackie Achmat.[281]

the lack of proper systems for monitoring
and follow-up care. Taking ARVs is problematic. Some 30% of people suffer severe side-
effects that include inflammation of the
pancreas and painful nerve damage. AZT
(Zidovudine; trade name: Retrovir) may also
cause a depletion of red or white blood
cells, especially when taken in the later
stages of the disease. Other common side-
effects associated with protease inhibitors
include nausea, diarrhoea and other gastro-
intestinal symptoms. In addition, protease
inhibitors can interact with other drugs,
resulting in serious-side effects. ARVs should
also be accompanied by good nutrition.

Poor adherence is a problem with chronic
medication in general and ARVs in particular. People may take their drugs erratically
or stop taking them altogether. For example,
the treatment for TB requires strict adherence to the treatment programme for a min-
imum of six months. This is not always successful. Drug supplies are sometimes erratic
and a number of patients stop taking the
drugs when they feel better. This compromises the health of the individual patient as
well as society as a whole because it leads to
drug-resistant strains of the virus. Drug-
resistant TB is now a huge problem in South
Africa as a direct result of non-adherence to
drug regimes.

HAART successfully reduces viral load to
undetectable levels in many people but viral
load rebounds quickly if the treatment is
stopped. Obviously the severe side-effects of
ARVs may lead to people not taking their
medication. Poor adherence is also not just a
problem in less wealthy communities, as is
often assumed, and it can compromise the
health of the current population and future
generations. Treatment literacy is thus a priority in the distribution and management of
chronic medication. The Directly Observable
Treatment System (DOTS) has been widely
used in Africa, with uneven results. Quite

simply, the system involves designated family or community members observing patients taking their medication on a regular and ongoing basis.

Another complication is the need to assess the effectiveness of ARVs over time. This involves regular blood tests to monitor viral load. In Brazil this particular problem was successfully overcome by the introduction of mobile laboratories. But South Africa does not have the capacity to administer and monitor the provision of ARVs in all parts of the country. Our health-care system reflects deep inequities, particularly between rural and urban areas. It would be possible to provide ARVs in major metropolitan centres such as Johannesburg or Cape Town. However, in rural areas that lack basic necessities such as drug supply systems and health personnel this would not be possible immediately. The health system would need to build on current capacity and make plans to improve capacity where it is absent. Inequities in the health-care system would therefore have to be tackled concurrently.

It is sometimes argued that government resources should be allocated to poverty reduction rather than expensive treatment regimes. But clearly there is a strong link between HIV/AIDS and poverty. Poor people are more vulnerable to HIV infection and people with AIDS live longer when they are better nourished. 'This is an argument for fighting AIDS and poverty – not for fighting poverty instead of treating AIDS. It is an argument for providing food parcels to poor people on ARVs (as happens in the Western Cape) – not an argument for providing food parcels only.'[282]

Luyanda is one of three AIDS orphans living with his granny in their Tembisa home after his mother died about three years ago. All four people are dependent on his grandmother's state pension. Although they have planted pumpkins in their garden to supplement their diet, Luyanda often goes to bed hungry. His application for a social grant was made two years ago.[283]

Shortly before Moses' mother died last year, she called her children to her one by one, to say goodbye. It was only during those final moments that she revealed she had AIDS. Her children nursed her until two days before her death, when she was taken to Mofolo Hospice. Moses (8), who is also HIV positive, faces a similar death. He is visibly smaller than his uninfected twin brother, his growth stunted as sometimes seen with infected children. His shoes are two sizes smaller than those of his twin. His application for a social grant has failed because he couldn't produce a birth certificate.[284]

WHAT IS TO BE DONE?

The AIDS epidemic is very complex. The virus itself has confounded the world's best scientists for over 20 years. At a point when science appeared to be invincible, and epidemics a thing of the past, AIDS has shaken faith in the capacity of medical research and technology. There is still no cure and no vaccine. However, it is likely that the extraordinary level of research into HIV will ultimately transform the face of medical science.

AIDS also magnifies social inequalities. This is starkly apparent in the Southern African region with its long history of inequality and dispossession. AIDS cannot be tackled effectively without addressing this historical legacy. We have argued throughout the book that AIDS must be understood as a social problem, not just a disease that affects individuals. Locating AIDS in context can make the obstacles seem insurmountable and the problems overwhelming. Some solutions are social. These range from poverty alleviation strategies to addressing basic infrastructural needs such as unemployment, education and housing.

In some instances measures are already in place that could alleviate poverty. But these are often inaccessible owing to bureaucratic rules and inefficiency. A stark example of this is that while AIDS orphans are entitled to social grants they often struggle to access them.

Children under the age of nine are entitled to R160 a month in child-support grants. Older children could access R500-a-month foster-care grants if the eldest sibling becomes a foster parent. But the so-called 'Primary Adult Care-giver' to whom child support grants are paid has to be aged at least 21 years, and older siblings are not allowed to become foster parents before the age of 21 either. This leaves many child-headed families out in the cold. One Tembisa household currently has sixteen AIDS orphans, four of whom are HIV infected, but none with social grants. The eldest is 20 years old.[285]

One of the problems is the extraordinarily long time that it takes to process social welfare grant applications. In some instances applicants are still waiting for a response three years on.

In some instances files are lost or the process of applying for grants is impeded by the need to produce birth certificates. One study showed that lack of financial resources and an inability to access state grants such as child support are the most consistent problems elderly women caregivers face. This is largely because of the bureaucracy involved in doing so. The absence of documentation such as birth and death certificates and identity documents (of the grandparents themselves, their children and grandchildren) prevents them from applying for and receiving state support. This is in line with other research conducted in the region where it has been found that as many as 70% of children in some areas do not have birth certificates.[286]

A simple matter like the lack of documentation can be a life-and-death issue, but is easily remedied. It is also possible to improve other strategies such as voluntary testing and counselling. Early diagnosis allows for the possibility of early treatment, including that of opportunistic infections.

Because it is sexually transmitted, AIDS evokes cultural taboos, fears and beliefs about sex. Sexuality is closely linked to individual psychology and personal identity. Trying to change sexual behaviour carries the risk of exposing an intimate realm of human life. So interventions need to confront all the fears, taboos, desires and passions associated with sexuality. The epidemic is hard to understand and hard to stop. Yet it is clear that people are slow to change their sexual behaviour. In the short term, the factors that prevent a dramatic change in sexual practices are daunting.

Ultimately HAART is the only treatment option currently available for people with AIDS. This is notwithstanding the challenge of implementation arising from an inefficient and under-resourced health-care system and the problems of drug compliance. If we are to provide treatment for other chronic diseases that are preventable, for example diabetes and hypertension, we are obligated to do the same for HIV. HAART has dramatically reduced mortality in countries that have made the drug available (including developing countries such as Brazil and Thailand). It should thus be made freely and immediately available in areas that have the health-care infrastructure to do so. Capacity must be improved in other areas allowing for an incremental implementation strategy. The health-care programme must include comprehensive Mother-to-Child Transmission Prevention Programmes (MTCTPs), as well as aggressive treatment of STIs and AIDS-related opportunistic infections. It must be complemented with improved access to welfare, such as child-support grants. It should also include on-going social programmes aimed at combating domestic violence and child abuse and promoting behavioural and relationship change. AIDS should be the most important political priority in the region.

ENDNOTES

INTRODUCTION

1 AIDS has also been said to stand for 'Afrikaner Invention to Deprive us of Sex' (Van der Vliet 2001:155)

2 United Nations Office for the Coordination of Humanitarian Affairs, fourth general assembly of the African Population Commission, 12 February 2002.

3 *The Independent*, 10 February 2000.

4 www.suntimes.co.za/2000/07/09.

5 health-e, 27 July 2001.

6 www.suntimes.co.za/2000/07/16.

7 Interview by Kerry Cullinan, www.suntimes.co.za/2001/11/25.

8 Dorrington *et al.*, 2001:1.

9 Walker and Gilbert, 2002; Marks, 2002; Skordis and Nattrass, 2001.

10 Bloom and Godwin, 1997.

11 Marks, 2002:15.

12 www.suntimes.co.za/2000/07/16.

13 Van der Vliet, 2001:153.

14 Edwin Cameron, Conference Address, 13th International AIDS Conference, Durban, 2000, www.suntimes.co.za/2000/07/16/insight/

1   SEX AND POWER IN SOUTH AFRICA

15 Barnett and Whiteside, 2002:154.

16 Ibid:153.

17 Foreman, 1999:viii.

18 Jewkes, 2001:1.

19 Wood and Jewkes, 1997:42.

20 Becker, 2001:7.

21 Derogatory term, usually applied to a single mother, denoting 'loose woman' and often translated as 'bitch'. Ibid:8.

22 Nduna *et al.*, 2001:7-8.

23 Ibid:8.

24 Gear, 2001:6.

25 Ibid:8.

26 Niehaus, 2002:24.

27 Skinner, 2001:5.

28 Ibid:5.

29 Collins and Stadler, 2001:5.

30 Ibid:4.

31 Nduna *et al.*, 2001.

32 Pattman, 2001:17.

33 Hunter, 2002:107.

34 Thorpe, 2001.

35 *Homeless Talk*, May 2002.

36 Nduna *et al.*, 2001:7.

37 Ashforth, 1999:51.

38 Wood, forthcoming

39 Nduna *et al.*, 2001:9.

40 Becker, 2001:12.

41 Leclerc-Madlala, 2000:28-29.

42 Thorpe, 2001:8.

43 Mlungwana, 2001:9.

44 Niehaus, 2002.

45 Becker, 2001.

46 Ibid:13.

47 Pattman, 2001.

48 Thorpe, 2001:8.

49 Niehaus, 2002.

50 Interview conducted by Mpumi Njinge at Springs station. Source: *My Son the Bride*. Video Documentary, 2002, directed by Mpumi Njinge.

51 Collins and Stadler, 2001.

52 Ibid:6.

53 Ibid:7.

54 Marcus, 2001:5.

55 Thorpe, 2001:8.

56 Skinner, 2001:8.

57 Thorpe, 2001:13.

58 Collins and Stadler, 2001:4.

59 Ibid:5.

60 Marcus, 2001:7.

61 Skinner, 2001:8.

62 Thorpe, 2001:7.

63 Collins and Stadler, 2001:5.

64 Niehaus, 2002.

65 Niehaus, 2002:25.

66 Ibid:25.

67 Hoosen and Collins, 2001.

68 Malala, 2001.

69 Skinner, 2001:7.

70 Thorpe, 2001:6.

71 Skinner, 2001:6.

72 Epprecht, 2001; Niehaus, 2002:28.

73 Foreman, 1999.

74 Reid and Dirsuweit, 2002.

75 Caronavo, 1995:5.

76 Achmat, 1999.

77 Jewkes, 2001:1.

78 Ntlabati *et al.*, 2001.

79 Foreman, 1999:7.

80 Ntlabati *et al.*, 2001:10.

81 Ibid:10.

82 Hoosen and Collins, 2001:12.

83 Pattman, 2001:18.

84 Hoosen and Collins, 2001:13.

85 Shabalala, 2001:5.

86 Hunter, 2002:111.

87 Ibid:112.

88 Ibid:114.

89 Ibid:114.
90 Ibid:113.
91 Leggett, 2001.
92 Ibid:100-105.
93 Ibid:110.
94 Williams *et al.*, 2000.
95 Leggett, 2001:110.
96 Hoosen and Collins, 2001:11.
97 Leggett, 2001:103.
98 Ntlabati *et al.*, 2001.
99 Ibid:14.
100 Ibid:11.
101 Hoosen and Collins, 2001:11.
102 Ibid:11.
103 Foreman, 1999:72.
104 Leclerc-Madlala, 2001:3.
105 Hoosen and Collins, 2001:9.
106 Gilbert and Walker, 2002:1098.
107 Stadler, 2001:18.
108 Ibid:13.
109 Shabalala, 2001:5.
110 Marais, 2000 53.
111 Collins and Stadler, 2001:1-2.
112 Ronnie Govender, *Sunday Times*, 6 October 2002.
113 Sideris (in Hammond), 1998:30.
114 Delius and Glaser, 2002.
115 *Mail & Guardian*, 25 Jan 2002.
116 *The Star*, 4 March 2001.
117 Ntlabati *et al.*, 2001.
118 Jewkes, 2001.
119 Hlongwa, 2001.
120 Van der Riet, 2001.
121 Hunter, 2001.
122 *Mail & Guardian*, 8 March 2002.
123 Gear, 2001.
124 Peltzer, cited in Nduna *et al.*, 2001.
125 Van der Riet, 2001.
126 Collins and Stadler, 2001.
127 Nduna *et al.*, 2001:7.
128 Leclerc-Madlala, 2000:29.
129 Collins and Stadler, 2001.
130 Thorpe, 2001:6.
131 AREPP Educational Trust, 2001:9.
132 Ndlovu and Ngwenya, 2001.
133 Denis and Makiwane, 2001:6.

2   'AN EPIDEMIC WAITING TO HAPPEN'

134 The chapter heading is the title of Shula Marks's address to the AIDS in Context Conference, published in *African Studies*, 61(1), 2002.
135 Kark, cited in Marks, 2002:18.
136 Delius, 1996:23.
137 Campbell, 1997:277-78.
138 Breckenridge, 1998:669-94.
139 Guy and Thabane, 1988:258-78; Bonner, 1992:269-305.
140 Beinart, 1991:103-28; Breckenridge, 1998:677-78.
141 Delius, 1996:25.
142 Moodie, 1994.
143 Niehaus, 2002:82.
144 Jochelson, 2003:12-16.
145 Bonner, 1990a.
146 Mager, 1999:87.
147 Ibid.
148 Mager, 1999:128.
149 Bonner, 1990b:229.
150 For one notable example see Bonner, 1993:160-94.
151 Williams *et al.*, 2000.
152 Lurie, 2000:344.
153 Bonner and Nieftagodein, 2001:54.
154 Ibid:56.
155 Barnett and Whiteside, 2002:151.
156 Marks, 2002:18.
157 Jeeves, 2001.
158 Lurie, 2000:345-46.
159 Packard and Coetzee, cited in Horwitz, 2001:1.
160 Williams, cited in Williams *et al.*, 1997:132.
161 Horwitz, 2001:16.
162 Delius, 1996:35.
163 Marks, 2002:16.
164 H. Phillips, 2001:10.
165 Department of Health, Health Systems Research Coordination and Epidemiology Directorate, June 2000
166 McKeown, 1979.
167 Jeeves, 2001:10.
168 www.sahealthinfo.org/publications/tbburden.htm
169 Putnam *et al.*, cited in Harriss and De Renzio, 1997:920.
170 See for example, Hawe and Shiell, 2000:871-85.
171 Jeeves, 2001:6.
172 Ibid:5.
173 *Mail & Guardian*, 26 October 2001.
174 H. Phillips, 2001:4.
175 Jeeves, 2001:7.
176 Hunter, 2001:15-16.
177 Delius and Glaser, 2002.
178 Delius and Glaser, 2002:30.
179 Ntlabati *et al.*, 2001:15.
180 Horwitz, 2001:12.
181 Carton, cited in Delius and Glaser, 2002:33.
182 Delius and Glaser, 2002:36.
183 Mayer, cited in Delius and Glaser, 2002:37.
184 Delius and Glaser, 2002:42.
185 Hellmann and Longmore, cited in Delius and Glaser, 2002:46.
186 Delius and Glaser, 2002.
187 Dorrington, 2001:11.
188 Hoosen and Collins, 2001:15.
189 Crewe, 1992:56.
190 Marks, 2002:19.

191 Beinart, 2001:314.
192 May, 1998:6.
193 Poswell, 2002:4.
194 May, 1998:82.
195 Beinart, 2001:277.
196 Sapire, 1992:673-76.
197 Marks, 2002:19.
198 Glaser, 2000.
199 Grundlingh, 2001:5.
200 Crewe, 1992:57.
201 Schneider, 2002:147.

3   CULTURAL COLLISIONS
202 Wolf, 2001:2.
203 Fadiman, 1997.
204 Heald, 2002:1.
205 Ibid:1.
206 Mlungwana, 2001:4.
207 Malala, 2001:4.
208 Thornton, 2002:10.
209 Clarke, E (1998) www.hst.org.za/update/37/
     policy5.htm, October 1998.
210 Pretorius, 1999:1.
211 Thornton, 2002:15.
212 Reuther, 2001:5.
213 Thornton, 2002:23.
214 Comaroff 1985:83.
215 Dilger, 2001:16.
216 Thabo Mohlala, *Mail & Guardian*, 30 November
     2001.
217 Heald, 2002:3.
218 Ibid:4.
219 Ibid:4.
220 Ibid:4.
221 Ibid:5.
222 Ibid:6.
223 Ibid:6.
224 Wolf, 2001:1.
225 Ibid:2.
226 Ibid:2.
227 Ibid:5.
228 Baez *et al.*, 2001:28.
229 Thornton, 2002:26.
230 Ibid:27.
231 Ibid:28.
232 Ibid:28.
233 Ibid:30.
234 Malala, 2001:5.
235 Dilger, 2001:16.
236 Ashforth, 2002:126.
237 Ibid:128.
238 Ibid:129–30.
239 Ibid:134.
240 Stadler, 2001:14.
241 Thokozani Mtshali, *Sunday Times*, 28 April 2002.
242 Stadler, 2001:13.

243 Shabalala, 2001:6.
244 Ibid:10.
245 Nzokia 2000:11.
246 Crewe, 1992:61.
247 B. Horner, *Sunday Times*, 6 October 2002.
248 Heald, 2002:8.
249 Scorgie, 2002:68.

4   CONFRONTING THE EPIDEMIC
250 Cameron, 2001:15.
251 Ibid:15.
252 O. Phillips, 2001:8.
253 Karim, cited in Schneider, 2002:161.
254 *Sunday Times*, 15 April 2001.
255 Figueira, 2001:19.
256 Berger, 2001.
257 Garson, 1994.
258 Schneider, 2002:163.
259 Ibid:164.
260 James, 2002:180.
261 Ibid:172.
262 Ibid:180.
263 Tallis, cited in James, 2002:184.
264 Kelly and Parker, 2001:2.
265 Walker and Reid, 2002.
266 Ibid:6.
267 Stadler, 2001.
268 Ibid.
269 Pronyk *et al.*, 2001:10.
270 Stadler, 2001:14.
271 See the box on page 121.
272 Satcher, cited in Pronyk *et al.*, 2001:6.
273 N. Nattrass, *Saturday Star*, 9 February 2003.
274 Ibid.
275 Macintyre, cited in Kelly and Parker, 2001:1.
276 Cameron, 2001:5.
277 Schneider, 2002:150.
278 Ibid:153.
279 Nattrass, 2003b.
280 Cameron, cited in Berger, 2001:2.
281 *Business Day*, 27 September 2002.
282 Nattrass, 2003b.
283 *The Star*, 30 April 2003.
284 Ibid.
285 Ibid.
286 Ferreira *et al.*, 2001.

BIBLIOGRAPHY

Achmat, Z. (1999). We Mourn Simon Tseko Nkoli. *Equality*, Issue 4, June.

AREPP Educational Trust. (2001). Documenting HIV/AIDS Good Practices in South Africa. Report presented at the AIDS in Context Conference, 4–7 April, University of the Witwatersrand, Johannesburg.

Ashforth, A. (1999). Weighing Manhood in Soweto. *CODESRIA Bulletin*, 3 & 4.

Ashforth, A. (2002). An Epidemic of Witchcraft? *African Studies*, 61(1).

Baez, C., Manzana, M. and Moleme, M. (2001). Knowledge, Attitudes and Practices of Traditional Birth Attendants in Lejweleputsoa Health District. Paper presented at the AIDS in Context Conference, 4–7 April, University of the Witwatersrand, Johannesburg.

Barnett, T. and Whiteside, A. (2002). *AIDS in the Twenty-First Century*. Hampshire: Palgrave Macmillan.

Becker, H. (2001). I am the Man. Historical and Contemporary Perspectives on Masculinities in Northern Namibia. Paper presented at the AIDS in Context Conference, 4–7 April, University of the Witwatersrand, Johannesburg.

Beinart, W. (1991). The Origins of the *Indlabini* Male Associations and Migrant Labour in the Transkei. *African Studies*, 50(1 & 2).

Beinart, W. (2001). *Twentieth Century South Africa*. Oxford: Oxford University Press.

Berger, J. (2001). Tripping over Patents: International Trade, Compulsory Licences and Essential Treatments for HIV. Paper presented at the AIDS in Context Conference, 4–7 April, University of the Witwatersand, Johannesburg.

Bloom, D. & Godwin, P. (1997). The Economics of HIV/AIDS. Cited in briefing document *The Impact of HIV on Local Government and INCA's Sphere of Business* (2001), prepared by L. Thomas, C. Marx, M. Crewe, L. Walker, A. van der Heever and U. Bleibaum.

Bonner, P.L. (1990a). African Urbanisation on the Rand between the 1930s and 1940s: Its Social Character and Political Consequence. *Journal of Southern African Studies*, 21(1).

Bonner, P.L. (1990b). Desirable or Undesirable Basotho Women? Liquor, Prostitution and the Migration of Basotho Women to the Rand, 1920–1945. In C. Walker (ed.) *Women and Gender in South Africa to 1945*. Cape Town: David Philip.

Bonner, P.L. (1992). Backs to the Fence: Law, Liquor and the Search for Social Control in an East Rand Town, 1929-42. In J. Crush and C. Ambler (eds.) *Liquor and Labour in Southern Africa*. Ohio: Ohio University Press.

Bonner, P.L. (1993). The Russians on the Reef: Urbanisation, Gang Warfare, and Ethnic Mobilisation, 1947–1957. In P.L Bonner, P. Delius and D. Posel (eds.) *Apartheid's Genesis, 1934–1962*. Johannesburg: Ravan Press.

Bonner, P. and Nieftagodein, N. (2001). *Kathorus. A History*. Cape Town: Maskew Miller Longman.

Breckenridge, K. (1998). The Allure of Violence: Men, Race and Masculinity on the South African Gold Mines, 1900–1950. *Journal of Southern African Studies*, 24(4).

Business Day (27 September 2002). Government can avoid 3 million AIDS deaths.

Cameron, E. (2001). Opening Address. AIDS in Context Conference, 4–7 April, University of the Witwatersrand, Johannesburg.

Campbell, C. (1997). Migrancy, Masculine Identities and AIDS: The Psychosocial Context of HIV Transmission on the South African Gold Mines. *Social Science and Medicine*, 42(2).

Caronavo, K. (1995). HIV and the Challenges Facing Men. *Issues Paper 15*, HIV and Development Programme. New York: UNDP/Kumarian.

Collins, T. and Stadler, J. (2001). Love, Passion and Play: Sexual Meaning among Youth in the Northern Province of South Africa. Paper presented at the AIDS in Context Conference, 4–7 April, University of the Witwatersrand, Johannesburg.

Comaroff, J. (1985). *Body of Power, Spirit of Resistance*. Chicago: University of Chicago Press.

Cornell, M. (2001). AIDS in Context. Unpublished conference report.

Crewe, M. (1992). *AIDS in South Africa*. London: Penguin.

Delius, P. (1996). *A Lion amongst the Cattle*. Johannesburg: Ravan Press.

Delius, P and Glaser, C. (2002). Sexual Socialisation in South Africa: A Historical Perspective. *African Studies*, 61(1).

Denis, P. and Makiwane, N. (2001). Oral History in the Context of AIDS: Memory Boxes as a Way of Building up Resilience in Orphans and Traumatised Children in KwaZulu-Natal. Paper presented at the AIDS in Context Conference, 4–7 April, University of the Witwatersrand, Johannesburg.

Dilger, H. (2001). Living Positively in Tanzania: The Global Dynamics of AIDS and the Meaning of Religion for International and Local AIDS Work. Paper presented at the AIDS in Context Conference, 4–7 April, University of the Witwatersrand, Johannesburg.

Dorrington, R. (2001a). The Demographic Impact of HIV/AIDS in South Africa by Province, Race and Class. Paper presented to the AIDS in Context Conference, 4–7 April, University of the Witwatersrand, Johannesburg.

Dorrington, R., Bourne, D., Bradshaw, D., Laubscher, R. and Timaeus, I. (2001). *The Impact of HIV/AIDS on Adult Mortality in South Africa, Technical Report, Burden of Disease Research Unit.* Cape Town: Medical Research Council.

Drum. (February 1991). Is AIDS a conspiracy against Blacks?

Epprecht, M. (2001). *Umteto ka sokisi:* 'The Rules of Mine Marriage' and the Sexual Content of Male-Male Sexual Relationships in Early 20th-Century Southern Africa. Paper presented at the AIDS in Context Conference, 4–7 April, University of the Witwatersrand, Johannesburg.

Fadiman, A. (1997). *The Spirit Catches You and You Fall Down. A Hmong Child, Her American Doctors, and the Collision of Two Cultures.* New York: Farrar, Straus and Giroux.

Ferreira, M., Keikelame M.J. and Mosaval, Y. (2001). *Older Women as Carers to Children and Grandchildren Affected by AIDS: A Study towards Supporting the Carers.* Institute of Ageing in Africa, Faculty of Health Sciences, University of Cape Town.

Figueira, M. (2001). HIV/AIDS: Human Rights Developments in Namibia since Independence. Paper presented at the AIDS in Context Conference, 4–7 April, University of the Witwatersrand, Johannesburg.

Foreman, M. (1999). *Men and AIDS: Taking Risks, Taking Responsibility.* London: Zed Press.

Garson, P. (1994). The AIDS Kaffirs of Johannesburg Prison. *Mail & Guardian,* 29 July.

Gear, S. (2001). Sex, Sexual Violence and Coercion in Men's Prisons. Paper presented at the AIDS in Context Conference, 4–7 April, University of the Witwatersrand, Johannesburg.

Gevisser, M. (2001). From Blood to Sweat and Tears, www.sundaytimes.co.za/2001/04/15/insight/in03.htm.

Gilbert, L. and Walker, L. (2002). 'Treading the Path of Least Resistance'. HIV/AIDS and Social Inequality and HIV/AIDS – A South African Case Study. *Social Science and Medicine,* 54.

Glaser, C. (2000). *Bo-Tsotsi: The Youth Gangs of Soweto 1935–1976.* Portsmouth: Heinemann.

Govender, R. (2002). AIDS takes its toll in infant mortality. Hundreds of tiny coffins bear witness to the extent of fatal disease. *Sunday Times,* 6 October.

Grundlingh, L. (2001). A Critical Historical Analysis of Government Responses to HIV/AIDS in South Africa as Reported in the Media, 1983–1994. Paper presented at the AIDS in Context Conference, 4–7 April, University of the Witwatersrand, Johannesburg.

Guy, J. and Thabane, M. (1988). Technology, Ethnicity and Ideology: Basotho Miners and Shaft Sinking on the South African Gold Mines. *Journal of Southern African Studies,* 14(4).

Hammond, S. (1998). African Eye News Service.

Harriss, J. and De Renzio, P. (1997). An Introductory Bibliographic Essay, *Journal of International Development,* 9(7).

Hawe, P. and Shiell, A. (2000) Social Capital and Health Promotion: A Review. *Social Science and Medicine,* 51.

Heald, S. (2002). It's Never as Easy as ABC: Understandings of AIDS in Botswana. *African Journal of AIDS Research,* 1(1).

Hlongwa, L (2001). Comparing the Lifestyle of Urban and Rural Youth: A Case Study of Two Schools in KwaZulu-Natal. Paper presented at the AIDS in Context Conference, 4–7 April, University of the Witwatersrand, Johannesburg.

Hoosen, S. and Collins, A. (2001). Women, Culture and AIDS: How Discourses of Gender and Sexuality Affect Safe Sex Behaviour. Paper presented at the AIDS in Context Conference, 4–7 April, University of the Witwatersrand, Johannesburg.

Horwitz, S. (2001). History, Migrancy and Patterns of Disease. Paper presented at the AIDS in Context Conference, 4–7 April, University of the Witwatersrand, Johannesburg.

Hunter, M. (2001). The Ambiguity of AIDS 'Awareness' and the Power behind Forgetting: Historicizing and Spatializing Inequality in Mandeni, KwaZulu-Natal. Paper presented at the AIDS in Context Conference, 4–7 April, University of the Witwatersrand, Johannesburg.

Hunter, M. (2002). The Materiality of Everyday Sex: Thinking beyond 'Prostitution'. *African Studies*, 61(2).

James, D. (2002). 'To Take the Information down to the People': Life Skills and HIV/AIDS, Peer Educators in the Durban Area. *African Studies*, 61(1).

Jeeves, A. (2001). Public Health and Epidemiology in the Era of South Africa's VD Pandemic of the 1930s and 1940s. Paper presented at the AIDS in Context Conference, 4–7 April, University of the Witwatersrand, Johannesburg.

Jewkes, R. (2001). Gender-based Violence, Gender Inequalities and the HIV Epidemic. Paper presented at the AIDS in Context Conference, 4–7 April, University of the Witwatersrand, Johannesburg.

Jochelson, K. (2003). *The Colour of Disease: Syphilis and Racism in South Africa, 1880–1950*. Oxford: Palgrave.

Kelly, K. and Parker, W. (2001). From People to Places: Prioritising Contextual Research for Social Mobilisation against HIV/AIDS. Paper presented at the AIDS in Context Conference, 4–7 April, University of the Witwatersrand, Johannesburg.

Leclerc-Madlala, S. (2000). The silence that nourishes AIDS in Africa. *Mail & Guardian*, 11–17 August.

Leclerc-Madlala, S. (2001). The ABCs of Virginity. *WHP Review: The Quarterly Journal of Women's Health Project*, 40.

Leggett, T. (2001). *Rainbow Vice. The Drugs and Sex Industries in the New South Africa*. Cape Town: David Philip.

Lurie, M. (2000). Migration and AIDS in Southern Africa: A Review. *South African Journal of Science*, 96.

Mager, A. (1999). *Gender and the Making of a South African Bantustan: A Social History of the Ciskei, 1945–1959*. Oxford: James Currey.

Malala, J. (2001). Perceptions of the Body, Illness and Disease amongst Sex Workers in Hillbrow. Paper presented at the AIDS in Context Conference, 4–7 April, University of the Witwatersrand, Johannesburg.

Marais, H. (2000). *To the Edge: AIDS Review 2000*. Pretoria: Centre for the Study of AIDS, University of Pretoria.

Marcus, T. (2001). Kissing the Cobra: Sexuality and High Risk in a Generalised Epidemic: A Case Study. Paper presented at the AIDS in Context Conference, 4–7 April, University of the Witwatersrand, Johannesburg.

Marks, S. (2002). An Epidemic Waiting to Happen. *African Studies*, 61(1).

May, J. (1998). *Poverty and Inequality in South Africa*. Report prepared for the Office of the Executive Deputy President and the Inter-Ministerial Committee for Poverty and Inequality. Government Communications.

McKeown, T. (1979). *The Role of Medicine*. Oxford: Blackwell.

Mlungwana, J. (2001). Cultural Dilemmas in Life Skills Education in KZN: Umbonambi Primary School Project. Paper presented at the AIDS in Context Conference, 4–7 April, University of the Witwatersrand, Johannesburg.

Mohlala, T. (2001). Turning to traditional healers. *Mail & Guardian*, 30 November.

Moleleki, J. (2002). I never gave her a smile. *Homeless Talk*, May.

Moodie, T.D. (1994). *Going for Gold: Mines, Men and Migration*. Berkeley: University of California Press.

Mtshali, T. (2002). I have seen my family die of AIDS but no one believes it. *Sunday Times*, 28 April.

Nattrass, N. (2003a). HIV drugs will save money as well as lives. *Saturday Star*, 9 February.

Nattrass, N. (2003b). We need to fight AIDS *and* poverty. *Mail & Guardian*, 20 March 2003.

Ndlovu, D. and Ngwenya, S. (2001). Establishment of Options for Orphans: The Bushbuckridge Professional Foster Care Project. Paper presented at the AIDS in Context Conference, 4–7 April, University of the Witwatersrand, Johannesburg.

Nduna, N., Jama, N. and Jewkes, R. (2001). Stepping Stones: Preliminary Findings. Paper presented at the AIDS in Context Conference, 4–7 April, University of the Witwatersrand, Johannesburg.

Niehaus, I. (2002). Renegotiating Masculinity in the South African Lowveld: Narratives of Male–Male Sex in Labour Compounds and in Prisons. *African Studies*, 61(1).

Ntlabati, P., Kelly, K. and Mankayi, A. (2001). The First Time: An Oral History of Sexual Debut in a Deep Rural Area. Paper presented at the AIDS in Context Conference, 4–7 April, University of the Witwatersrand. Johannesburg.

Nzokia, C. (2000) The social meanings of death from HIV/AIDS: an African interpretative view. *Journal of Culture, Health and Society*, 2(1).

Pattman, (2001). Researching Student Identities and Addressing AIDS in Institutions of Higher Education in Southern Africa. Paper presented at the AIDS in Context Conference, 4–7 April, University of the Witwatersrand, Johannesburg.

Phillips, H. (2001). AIDS in the Context of South Africa's Epidemic History: Some Preliminary Thoughts. Paper presented at the AIDS in Context Conference, 4–7 April, University of the Witwatersrand, Johannesburg.

Phillips, O. (2001). Local Rights and the Legal Subject in a Global Context: Getting Access to Treatment. Paper presented to the AIDS in Context Conference, 4–7 April, University of the Witwatersrand, Johannesburg.

Poswell, L. (2002). *The Post-Apartheid South African Labour Market: A Status Report.* Cape Town: Development Policy Research Unit, University of Cape Town.

Pretorius, E. (1999). Traditional Healers. *South African Health Review.* Durban: Health Systems Trust.

Pronyk, P.M., Hargreaves, J.R., Kim, J.C. and Makhubele, M.B. (2001). Generating Social Capital through Micro-finance: The Design of a Multi-level HIV Prevention and Control Strategy. Paper presented at the AIDS in Context Conference, 4–7 April, University of the Witwatersrand, Johannesburg.

Putnam, R., Leonardi, R and Nanetti, R.Y. (1993). *Making Democracy Work: Civic Traditions in Modern Italy.* Princeton, NJ: Princeton University Press.

Reid, R. and Dirsuweit, T. (2002). Understanding Systemic Violence: Homophobic Attacks in Johannesburg and its Surrounds. *Urban Forum,* 13(3).

Reuther, K. (2001). AIDS and Healers in the South African Press: More of an Open Controversy Still Needed. Paper presented at the AIDS in Context Conference, 4–7 April, University of the Witwatersrand, Johannesburg.

Sapire, H. (1992). Politics and Protest in Shack Settlements of the Pretoria-Witwatersrand-Vereeniging Region, South Africa, 1980–1990. *Journal of Southern African Studies,* 18(3).

Schneider, H. (2002). On the Fault-line: The Politics of AIDS Policy in Contemporary South Africa. *African Studies,* 61(1).

Scorgie, F. (2002). Virginity Testing and the Politics of Sexual Responsibility: Implications for AIDS Intervention. *African Studies,* 61(1).

Shabalala, T.S. (2001). Once You Reveal that You are HIV Positive They Only See You as the Virus Itself: Experiences of Women Living with HIV/AIDS in Gauteng Province, South Africa. Paper presented at the AIDS in Context Conference, 4–7 April, University of the Witwatersrand, Johannesburg.

Skinner, D. (2001). How the Youth in Two Communities Make Decisions about Using Condoms. Paper presented at the AIDS in Context Conference, 4–7 April, University of the Witwatersrand, Johannesburg.

Skordis, J. and Natrass, N. (2001). What is Affordable: The Political Economy of Policy on the Transmission of HIV/AIDS from Mother to Child in South Africa. Paper presented at the AIDS in Context Conference, 4–7 April, University of the Witwatersrand, Johannesburg.

Stadler, J. (2001). 'He has a Heart of Listening': Reflections on a Community-based Care and Support Programme for People Infected with HIV/AIDS. Paper presented at the AIDS in Context Conference, 4–7 April, University of the Witwatersrand, Johannesburg.

Thornton, R. (2002). Traditional Healers, Medical Doctors and HIV/AIDS in Gauteng and Mpumalanga Provinces, South Africa. Draft report (unpublished).

Thorpe, M. (2001). Shifting Discourse: Teenage Masculinity and the Challenge for Behavioural Change. Paper presented at the AIDS in Context Conference, 4–7 April, University of the Witwatersrand, Johannesburg.

Van der Riet, M. (2001). Embedding Sexual Practice in Communities of Practice: The Contribution of Activity Theory. Paper presented at the AIDS in Context Conference, 4–7 April, University of the Witwatersrand, Johannesburg.

Van der Vliet, V., (2001). AIDS: Losing 'The New Struggle'? *Daedalus,* 130(1).

Walker, L. and Gilbert, L. (2002). HIV/AIDS: South African Women at Risk. *African Journal of AIDS Research,* 1(1).

Walker, L. and Reid, G. (2002). Aids and the Aged: Briefing Document. Unpublished report.

Williams, B.G., Campbell, C.M., MacPhail, C. (1997). The Carletonville Pilot Survey. In B. Williams, C. Campbell, C. Macphail (eds.) *Managing HIV/AIDS in South Africa. Lessons from Industrial Settings.* Braamfontein: CSIR.

Williams, B.G., Gilgen, D., Campbell, C.M., Taljaard, D. and MacPhail, C. (2000). *The Natural History of HIV/AIDS in South Africa: A Biomedical and Social Survey.* Braamfontein: Council for Scientific and Industrial Research (CSIR).

Wolf, A. (2001). AIDS or Kanyera? Concepts of Sexuality and the Discourse on Morality in Malawi. Paper presented at the AIDS in Context Conference, 4–7 April, University of the Witwatersrand, Johannesburg.

Wood, K. (forthcoming). Ethnographic Study of Sexual Health and Violence among Township Youth in the Eastern Cape, South Africa. Research data from PhD thesis, London School of Hygiene and Tropical Medicine.

Wood, K. and Jewkes, R. (1997). Violence, Rape and Sexual Coercion: Everyday Love in a South African Township. *Gender and Development,* 5.

INDEX

IMAGE CREDITS